DETOXIFICATION:

Powerful, Healthy Healing

By Dr. Elvis Ali, ND

ISBN:1539138186
ISBN: 13:9781539138181

DISCLAIMER

The information in this book are at all times restricted to education, teaching and training on the subject of natural health matters intended for general natural health wellbeing and do not involve the diagnosing, prognosticating, treatment, or prescribing of remedies for the treatment of any disease, or any licensed or controlled act which may constitute the practice of medicine.

Questions? Please email us at: drelvisali10@hotmail.com

CONTENTS

ACKNOWLEDGMENTS

It is a pleasure to acknowledge with thanks:

My entire family in Canada and Trinidad and Tobago who have continued to support and motivate me to educate others about naturopathic medicine. My parents, Hakim, Hazrah, my sisters, Alima, Homaida, Homeeda, Fazida, my children, Hassan, Azeeda, Kareem, Nephews, Nieces and precious grandchildren, Gursimran, Meheirveer and Shairveer for their encouragement and belief in holistic medicine.

Colleagues in the health care profession, especially Dr. Leo Roy.

My students and staff at CCNM, BINM, CCHH, OAND, CAND and clinics, BTNL, AA Comfort Health Centers and Mississauga clinic. The companies for their assistance in educating the public about preventative medicine, Biorrific, Ecoideas, Canadian Bio, Sangsters, Fion Beauty Supplies Canada, Alpha Science Laboratories – A division of Omega Alpha Pharmaceuticals Inc.

My dear friends, Bonita, Pat, Roy, Cindy and Darryl, Janak, Joan, Ash and Harry, Saira and Moe Sheikh of Etobicoke Motors along with many others too numerous to list.

My publisher and editor Sherree and Lillian who designed the book cover.

INTRODUCTION

When we hear the word detoxification we consider it to be a form of cruel punishment or deprivation. The thought of eating less or not eating for a while, and denying ourselves of the foods we love is absolutely cringe-worthy. Isn't it only for those with substance of alcohol abuse?

However, our bodies will thank us for giving them a time of rest from all the consumption of foods, drinks and substances we put in them on a daily basis. The body's organs are constantly working to keep it running efficiently. After a while, the organs become exhausted and cannot function at optimal levels anymore. When we start to feel sluggish, tired, unable to focus, even through the simplest mundane tasks, our body is in a toxic state.

In this book, I will be sharing the conditions that develop from a toxic body and the organs that are greatly affected. The main organ is the liver. The liver is actually the hardest working and most forgiving organ in our body. It is well known that the liver can repair and restore itself after years of abuse yet liver disease is the most chronic illness facing the world today. It is the third leading cause of death between the ages of 25 to 59. So you can imagine that it must be severe abuse to our body why the liver shuts down and people die.

Another organ is the gallbladder. What most people don't realize is how important the role of the gallbladder plays in assisting the liver to properly function. It produces the bile that helps the liver to release the toxins, but if the gallbladder doesn't produce enough bile, toxic wastes overload the liver and gallstones are the result. Most people remove gallstones, even their gallbladder without realizing that a change of eating habits and giving the body some respite may alleviate the discomfort and the gallstones will dissolve.

Another important consideration is the health of our gastrointestinal system. Constipation, a bloated stomach and passing excess gas are all symptoms of congested and toxic intestines.

Fasting is one of the most powerful ways of ridding the body of toxins. To not consume foods once a week, for a few days or a month or so, gives the body the opportunity to heal the right that is going wrong inside. Throughout the ages, a day of rest from eating was always considered beneficial for one's body and spirit.

When making the decision to fast, I highly recommend that you seek advice from your medical or holistic practitioner. It's very important that you know the state of your body to withstand a fast and for how long. Maybe all that is required is to drink freshly squeezed juices for a few hours a day without solids and at the end of the day have a light meal. There will most likely be pangs of hunger that gnaw at you, but sticking with it will certainly make a difference in reenergizing your body. Your body will love you for it!

CONSTIPATION: A Symptom not a Disease

Why a whole chapter on such a simple condition that merely requires a laxative to eliminate the problem?

Would it be so simple? Constipation is like an iceberg. Ninety percent of the problem escapes immediate observation. So many things that affect health, affect elimination.

To completely cure constipation requires a complete restoring of health.

Anything that adds to better living, improved vitality and to the general health of mind and body, not only helps correct constipation, but restores integrity to the whole body.

~~~~

There are some beliefs about eliminating body wastes and poisons that should be understood differently and appreciated more clearly in order to better achieve optimum health.

There are common misconceptions such as the following:

- It is considered normal to have one bowel movement a day.
- Only one bowel movement a day is necessary.
- It is quite all right to go several days without a bowl bowel movement.
- Such infrequent eliminations will never make you sick.

Facts: One bowel movement a day is <u>not</u> a normal and healthy habit. Every normal animal, living in the wilderness, will automatically have at least three bowel movements a day. Infants, as long as they are healthy – (health, meaning not just freedom from serious disease, but vital wellbeing) and well-nourished, have several bowel movements a day after being breastfed and/or eating natural foods.

Most adults who really care for their health - physically, emotionally and nutritionally, usually have a bowel elimination after every substantial meal eaten.

In our Western civilization there is a common acceptance to have one or less bowel movement on a daily basis. This acceptance is considered "average" which, in fact, is being confused with
~~~~

"normal". This is due to people living with questionable health and the universality of abnormal lifestyles, stresses, chemicals, artificial and processed foods.

It is more "normal" and obvious to believe that:

- Amounts of substances that go into the body must come out. If three substantial quantities of food are taken in each day, three bowel eliminations – an elimination of equal quantities should result.
- The buildup of residues and excesses of wastes and poisons retained in the body must eventually saturate the blood, the body fluids and the environment of cells. No cell can remain unaffected indefinitely. TOXICITY must inevitably become a health problem.
- For substances to be considered toxic, it is not essential that ill effects plague the body or be experienced immediately – within days, weeks or months. The accumulation and retention of anything that is not beneficial to cells, irritating, excessive, not in balance with the body's chemistry and needs, will inevitably produce a buildup of detrimental biochemical influences. These can be, and are over a period of time, as hazardous to health as taking doses of drugs or poisons which exert immediate harmful side effects.
- Simply taking a laxative to bring about bowel elimination is not an adequate answer. It is an over simplification. Laxatives are mostly stimulating. They can be whips. They whip the muscles of the intestinal tract into a contraction or spasm that paralyzes the normal intestinal flow brought on by its contraction/expansion (peristaltic movement) intestinal muscle action – called 'peristalsis'.
- Stimulation can improve the action of sluggish and tired intestinal muscles, but block elimination when these muscles are already too tense and in excess contraction.
- All laxatives are not harmless. Most commercial products are hazardous chemicals or drugs. They may be highly

effective in an emergency. They should not be taken repeatedly. Some can be habit forming.

- Herbal laxatives may not be as effective as the powerful drug forms in an emergency, but for anybody not in an acute crisis of disease, they are almost invariably, just as effective as drugs. They are harmless. They are not habit-forming – even if taken over a long period of time. To better understand the role of elimination – the 'when' and 'why 'of the need for laxatives for supplementary bowel flushing, it is essential to understand, beforehand, how the intestines function. Let us take a look.

The Intestines

The large and small intestine track consist of a resilient, hollow, hose-like tube, approximately 26 feet long that twists, turns and folds inside most of the lower abdomen.

Glands line the inner surface of the intestines. These glands secrete:

Enzymes are extremely important to the health of the intestines as well as for the whole body. They act on the foods coming down from the stomach. They break up the foods and prepare them for absorption, via the intestines into blood vessels which enmesh them. Without these enzymes, putrefaction and fermentation would occur. These toxic substances add to bowel irritation and constipation.

Mucus lubricates the inner surface. Mucus favors the normal flow of fecal matter.

The intestinal lining receives all of its nourishment, via arteries that transpierce the intestine muscles. Blood is the only source for nourishing and maintaining the health and functions of the glands that line the inner surface of the intestines.

Intestinal muscles surround and encircle the intestinal "tube" and produce the alternating contractions and expansion that push food and fecal matter through the length of the bowels. Excessive contractions (spasms) of the muscles may unduly constrict the blood circulation.

Peristalsis is the undulating flushing motion produced by the intestinal muscles can be: weak (sluggish), too slow or it can be over-stimulated, spasticity, hypertensive and contracted.

Tonus is the strength, the action, the efficiency and the normal state of contractibility of the muscles.

Factors that interfere with peristalsis are anything that is detrimental to the general health and hinder the normal functions of the intestines.

Causes of Constipation

The following depresses and weakens intestinal efficiency and makes the intestinal action sluggish.

- Malnutrition – an inadequate supply of the right foods and bulk.
- Deficiencies of much needed vitamins, minerals, enzymes and proteins.
- Negative emotions, exhaustion, depression, low morale and/or low self-image, and emotional repressions.
- Many drugs, chemicals and food additives.
- Fermentation: inaction and excessive decomposition of food.
- Excess intake together with inadequate digestion of foods.
- Inadequate provision of digestive enzymes of the saliva glands, stomach, pancreas and liver.
- Inadequate mastication and hasty gulping.
- Toxins and tensions are the main factors that inhibit peristalsis by overstimulation and/or paralysis. Toxins result from excessive lengthy retention of intestinal wastes and from...
- The intake of: irritating or poorly tolerated foods. Chemicals, preservatives, additives, colorings, pesticides, chemical fertilizers, pollutants and antibiotics etc., in foods.
- Drugs, chemicals and toxins with constipating side effects.

- Faulty digestion of foods. The undigested portions rot or ferment (known as putrefaction), and build up gases as toxic as drugs.
- Constipating foods, allergens, canned, overcooked and pasteurized foods.
- Diseases elsewhere in the body. Imbalanced glands, such as under active thyroid.
- Tensions include all forms of: stresses, anxieties, fears, envies, worries, frustrations, repressions of emotions, suppression of abilities and potentials.
- Faculty habits: the excesses of each person's lifestyle.

Atonic Constipation

Atonic constipation is bowel sluggishness – constipation from lack of muscle tone or strength. Extortion of the nerves and muscles of the intestines occur when the required levels of energy and nourishment are not adequate.

Nerve impulses become unable to stimulate the muscles and/or the muscles become too weak to contract and expand in their natural and essential stripping like evacuation movements.

Atonic constipation is recognized by changes in the elimination cycle and changes in the stools. Bowel movements are frequent, but large and bulky. Sometimes they are more dry and harder than normal. The stomach dilates. It protrudes. It looks like the early stage of obesity.

Exhaustion and malnutrition are the main and the responsible factors.

Excesses of that exhaustion:

- The bowels get as tired as does your whole body. While in exhaustion states – physical, mental, emotional – be they from play or work, drain energy from the bowels and inhibit their role.
- Poor sleep habits: Long night hours, agitated sleep, inadequate rest, holidays or relaxation.

- Years of straining and forcing to bring about bowel movements.
- Lack of exercise: excess inactivity also spells elimination disaster.
- Sedentary lifestyles: TV, immobility, prolonged desk work, poor posture - slumping. Confined to bed.

Foods that cause or increase Atonic constipation:

- Breads, including all foods which contain refined wheat and wheat flour.
- Cakes, cookies, biscuits, pies, dumplings, macaroni, spaghetti, sandwiches, dried boxed wheat serials, cream of wheat, etc.

Wheat flour thickens the bowels – makes them gluey. For many people, one slice of bread a day can inhibit one bowel movement a day.

- Pasteurized milk: boiled milk is an old remedy against diarrhea. The pasteurizing action is similar to that of boiling. It inhibits peristalsis – bowel elimination.
- Bulk-lacking foods: soft, mashed, overcooked foods, junk foods. Diets that is excessive in liquids. Excesses of juices, soups, jellies, puddings, starch foods, flower foods and all foods lacking their outer shells, skins, bran or coatings.

The colon needs bulk, which remains undigested and provides food for intestinal bacteria to flourish on.

Diet excesses: inadequate fibrous foods, inadequate fluids.

- Fat foods: pork, ham, bacon, sausages, canned tuna and salmon fishes. Fried foods, French fries, foods cooked with lard, shortening. Hot dogs, hamburgers, canned, processed meats. Cream, ice cream, margarine, other stale hydrogenated oils. Oils which have been heated and used for cooking. Don't reuse. Roasted or stale nuts. Nuts become stale when shells and skins are broken or gone and not speak, exposed to the air.

Fats block secretion of bile from the liver during meals bile is essential as a bowels stimulant – essential to soften fecal matter and to carry toxic matters out of the body.

- **High Salt Foods**: sea salt is only permissible in moderation. Table salt, salted butter, processed and most cheeses, seafood, fishes; canned, smoked, prepared meats and broths.
- **Drugs:** sedatives, tranquilizers, anesthetics and similar acting drugs. Opiates, pain relievers, hallucinogenic drugs and derivatives.
  - Antibiotics: destroy normal intestinal bacteria essential for a healthy bowel functioning.
  - Laxatives: prolong use brings on secondary exhaustion of intestines, resulting from excessive overstimulation. Mineral oil/Agarol-type laxatives. These dissolve and flush out oil soluble vitamins necessary for health of nerves, muscle physiologically physiology, calcium utilization and hormone formation.
- **Chemicals**: food additives, which destroy enzymes. All drugs do this. Foods lose enzymes on contact with air and heat, and when they go stale. The most potent enzyme destroyer are fluoride and its different compounds, including those currently found in drinking water, toothpastes, etc.
- Poisons from occupational hazards: Lead in paints, gas fumes, toxic chemicals contacted in industry, sometimes in the home. Aluminum products: cooking wearers, deodorants, aluminum is soluble in hot water and liquids.
- Aluminum compounds are nerve ending paralyzers (deodorants). Their action does not stop at poisoning the nerve endings which control perspiration through pores of

the skin. Their effects travel throughout all the nerves – those of the intestines and of the brain as well.

Many of the above products produce catarrh (increase of mucus) reactions in the bowels, as well as constipation. Many doctors have become heroes to their patients, just for curing their constipation by cutting them off some of this "57" varieties of drugs above.

- **Mental States**: negative attitude habits – chronic hopelessness and/or depressions.
- Negative attention to Nature's calls. The constant postponing of the passing of fecal matter. Excess stretching and dilating of muscles breakdown in their contracting ability.
- Chronic insomnia with exhaustion states; nervous breakdowns, etc.
- **Diseases:** shock states, be they from emotional trauma or surgery causes histamine to be released, which creates a ballooning affect of the colon.
- **Lack of Teeth**: mastication and food crushing are inadequate.
- **Hypothyroid:** this causes the most stubborn of all constipations. A poor thyroid brings on sluggish body function. It can be responsible for sluggish intestinal action with the consequence buildup of toxins, poor utilization of calcium by nerves and nerve fatigue.
- **Liver Congestion:** the liver's role is to detoxify and manufacture bile. Toxic buildup and lack of bile bring sluggishness of intestines and buildup of intestinal gases.
- **Intestinal Gas**: hinders normal growth of important intestinal bacteria. These beneficial bacteria creates Vitamins B1 and B12.
- **Chronic degenerative conditions and aging processes:** affect and slow down intestinal action as much as it does the body.

- **Prolapses of rectum, bladder, intestines or uterus:** Mechanical interference of normal intestinal peristalsis.
- **Posture habits and abdominal muscle weakness:** too much TV and desk sitting, lack of exercise and lack of proteins.
- **Anal fissures and hemorrhoids:** bring on reverse peristalsis.
- **Antibiotic intoxication:** they destroy essential bowel bacteria.
- **Deficiencies of vitamins and enzymes:** A, B, D, E, F.

Spastic Constipation: This is bowel constriction and or paralysis.

The nervous system can over activate the muscles of the intestines into a constricting contraction. Nerves, which are overactive or in a hyper-state, or nerves whipped into hyperactivity by chemical chemicals, tensions or other whips, may in turn, whip intestinal muscles into spasms. Spasms are contractions but don't fully release or relax.

The intestinal cavity cannot open adequately. Peristaltic waves are repressed. Fecal matter cannot be propelled along to the evacuation point.

Spastic intestines exists and are recognized when there is constipation accompanied by a state of general body uptightness or nervousness, tension, activity or by body toxicity. The inadequate passage of fecal matter takes the form of stools which are thin ribbons and/or small balls.

Some of the more specific factors which induce spastic constipation are:

- Tension inducing attitudes: the bowel becomes as tense as the rest of your body – as tense as you feel. The intestines react more strongly to tensions in a greater number of people than any other body organ.
- Selfishness: the mind that closes itself to others knows much tension. The tension overflows through the body and intestinal tenseness result.

- Anxieties, fears, angers, guilt, worries, repressions, holding back and holding things inside.
- Obsession: feeling obsessed by the need for a daily bowel movement and the obsessive use of laxatives is sufficient to tense up the bowels.
- Tensions inhibit or slow the production of saliva by the salivary glands. Saliva contains enzymes essential for the full digestion of starch and sugar type foods.
- Eating habits: overeating excess quantities and frequent snacks. For people to omit one meal a day is enough to effect a cure. Try this, if meals leave an uncomfortable stomach or bring on fatigue.
- Eating too fast: gulping down food, washing food down by drinking during meals; inadequate chewing.
- Eating when a previous meal has not been fully digested and the return of appetite has not signaled a further need for food.

Foods that contribute to spasticity constipation:

- Acid foods. Sugar in all forms and all foods that contain it: soft drinks, ice cream, candies, corn syrup and cornstarch. All boxed, processed cereals; grains without their outer shell and an excess of any grain. Many root vegetables without their skins.
- Over acidification of lower bowels by excesses of acid foods can notably interfere with maintaining normal health. Acid foods are strong stimulants. They unduly whip nerves.
- Allergens: foods in which a person is allergic will act like drugs.
- Fermenting and putrefying foods: inadequate digestion is responsible. Gases that form are practically as toxic as arsenic. Faulty digestion or intolerance to certain foods is recognized by the passing of gas either by mouth or rectum.
- Miscellaneous: alcohol and all alcoholic beverages baking powders and most spices and blackberries.

- Excessively cold foods: ice cold drinks, frozen foods and ice cream.

Toxins, drugs, chemicals that contribute to and cause spasticity constipation.

"Toxin" refers to all substances unnatural to the body's economy and health, and which are detrimental to cells and biochemical balance. These include:

- Undigested, unutilized and excess quantities of any foods.
- Undigested foods ferment or putrefy.
- Toxins and the buildup of acids from fermentation can be highly irritating to the colon. Materials in the colon must be alkaline at all times.

End products of abnormal body functioning and biochemical imbalances: all debris, broken down products and remnants of dying cells. Body chemicals created by fatigue, tensions, negative attitudes, etc. Waste products excreted by cells, damaged by injury, surgery or shock.

Guanidine: byproduct of putrefaction of proteins in the intestines. Infection poisons, such as drainage from abscesses in the body or in roots of teeth, from sinuses or from other sources of inflammation.

Allergens: chemicals or foods in which the body is intolerant or allergic. Unhealthy, stale, rotting, decaying, rancid foods (plant or animal); foodless, refined, processed, synthetic foods and food imitations.

Chemicals: all pollutants from the air, water and soil. Pesticides, chemical fertilizers and fumes from gases, oils (natural, propane, fuel gases), and cigarettes, etc.

Cosmetics: drug-type, deodorants, detergents, soaps and many toothpastes.

Food Additives: bleaching agents (such as in white flour, sugar foods), preservatives, sweeteners, emulsifiers, thickeners, thinners, coloring agents enriching vitamins and many more.

Drugs: stimulating type drugs, drug type laxatives, appetite suppressors, “Speed”.

Disease conditions that play a role in or cause’s spastic constipation:

- Overactive nervous system interacting and closely related to imbalances of the endocrine glands.
- Diseased organs, impacted wisdom teeth, tooth root abscesses.
- Spinal nerve root pressure from lordosis, scoliosis or vertebral deviations or misplacements.
- Inflammation, toxic states, abscesses of organs near to the intestines. Appendicitis, colitis, peritonitis or gallbladder problems.
- Pressures and/ or pinching of nerves or nerve branches. Old scars are common causes – scars that result from burns, surgery, cuts and inflammation. Nerves sometimes get caught in between the many fibers that come into the damaged area as part of the scar healing process. In the final stages of healing, these fibers can attach right onto nerve endings. Severe pinching irritates the nerves.
  The results can be intestinal spasm, inadequate functioning of the digestion organs: stomach, pancreas, liver and salivary glands.
- Deficiency diseases: the daily diet provides insufficient amounts of calcium, magnesium, vitamin-enzyme B and G complex, essential unsaturated oils and the vitamin – enzymes they contain.

Constipation Therapy

There is no ‘specific’ cure for constipation. How can there be since constipation is not a disease? It is a symptom – a warning sign, and alarm that indicates an impending breakdown of health somewhere in the body. It is always a result of some abnormality in body health or lifestyle.

Whatever diseases exist elsewhere in the body must always be considered and treated while correcting constipation. Often, these must be corrected first before constipation can be corrected.

To 'cure' constipation requires normalizing every pertinent aspect of health. The body's physiology must be healthy and balanced. Toxins must be eliminated. Energies must be restored. Health-giving habits must be incorporated into daily living. No cure is possible while one continues to persist in errors of living, faulty eating habits, continued intake of chemicals and abnormal foods.

There is no simple answer that can change, control or offset a life time of excesses and wrong habits. To alleviate only the symptoms of constipation is like setting up a smoke screen.

A quick review of causes listed above leaves little wonder that there can be no simple panacea or easy method for controlling or correcting so many factors that affect the intestines. Nor can one wonder that there are as many remedies for us for constipation as there are for colds.

Drugs and laxatives, as a cure, all are inadequate. They bypass the causes. To depend on these as an answer, can be gross negligence to healthcare.

Proper laxatives may be required temporarily. Diet, exercise and the elimination of all imbalances, hindrances and abnormalities must be a part of every constipation correction regime.

Laxative-acting Foods

An Herb Laxative Tea: in boiling spring water, brew the leaves from red raspberry and wild cherry plants, and bark from wild cherry or bayberry. Add a little honey to taste, if so desired.

Flax and Psyllium Seeds: soak in a cup full of either or both, until a jelly forms. Eat with a spoon. Add a little honey, if desired. Effectiveness increases when acidophilus yeast is added.

A Laxative Recipe: take 10 each of prunes, figs, apricots and dates. Mix them with four ounces of ginger root, a half a cup of honey and tablespoons of blackstrap molasses. Place in a sauce pan.

Brew one ounce of senna leaves in two cups of water. Add this water to the mixture in the saucepan. Let it stand and soak for 24 hours. Serve as stewed fruit. Eat a small plateful whenever constipated. Raisins, plums, peaches, apples and tomatoes can also be added.

Bulk-containing foods: skins, bran, coatings, polishing of vegetables and all grains; peas, beans, lentils and foods rich in cellulose: celery, leafy vegetables, cabbage and sauerkraut.
Always leave the skins on root vegetables. When you cook, do so lightly. Wrap in foil for baking or steam in waterless cookers.

All vegetables, including the root vegetables help constipation when they are not overcooked. During constipation, potatoes are best taken raw by grating and putting the gratings into lemon juice.

Whole sugar-type Foods: blackstrap molasses, whole fruits, natural honey. The effectiveness of honey as a laxative is best used for children. Mixing with lemon juice adds to the effect. Pasteurizing honey destroys laxative properties.

Juices: fruit and vegetable juices in moderation keep intestines lubricated. Use them when stools are dry and hard. Prune and cherry juices are best.

Salads: use any combination of green leafy vegetables. Delicious when served with raw cauliflower, asparagus, peas, apples, raisins and sunflower seeds. Add herbs and vegetable broth powders.

These foods are especially valuable when the stools are too acid. Use together with the skins of vegetables, fruits and grains, and mineral rich foods.

Mineral-rich foods: kelp, dulse, sea salt, vegetable broth powders, herbs, leafy vegetables. These supply both the gross and trace minerals. They increase food bulk. Serve by sprinkling generously on salads and in soups.

Whole Grains: grains are a rich source of phosphates and enzymes valuable in calcium utilization which improves nerve function and control. They are a principal source of acid reserves. They neutralize excess alkalinity of the bowels, which contributes to intestinal sluggishness.

Use rye, millet, flax, sesame seeds, oatmeal, buckwheat and some wheat, if desired. For cereals, add sunflower seeds and raisins. These last two, mixed with oatmeal, make an excellent raw cereal. Sweeten and make liquid by eating with a fruit juice – preferably pineapple.

For an ideal hot cereal, soak whole grains for 24 hours. Add raisins, sunflower seeds and oatmeal. Mix and soak in hot water. Don't cook or keep at a high temperature. Serve with butter and honey.

Oil Containing Foods: use especially when bowels are dry and hard. They lubricate the intestinal wall and eliminate the need for straining. The best of these are the following:

- **Internal organs**: liver, sweet breads; avocados and nuts when fresh and in shells.
- **Seed and grain oils**: sesame, flax and sunflower oils; Olive oil, soy and other oils when extracted without heat or chemicals can also be helpful. All oils must be fresh. Oils turn rancid quickly on contact with air and room temperature and heat. Never reuse heated oil. Rancid oils are constipating and detrimental to health.

Yogurt: that is made from unpasteurized, healthy milk. Yogurt, Kefir, lactic acid and acidophilus yeast help to regenerate essential, normal intestinal bacteria that is destroyed by antibiotics.

The Intestinal Bacteria: neutralize intestinal toxins and guanidine. They block the growth of undesirable bacteria in the intestines.

Fenugreek Tea: dissolves and flush mucous and catarrh from the intestines. Mucus can interfere with intestinal action when in excess. This tea also soothes irritated bowel walls and helps to lubricate the intestinal lining. If the taste is unpleasant, mix with other herb teas.

Dietary Advice for the Constipated:

- Avoid constipating foods. Review them on the previous pages.
- Eat foods in their uncooked, natural state whenever possible.
- For an effective persuader of bowel evacuation, drink daily on rising, a glass of warm lemon water. Use spring water, one teaspoon of lemon juice freshly squeezed and one teaspoon of honey.
- Make sure your diet contains plenty of bulk rich foods. However, avoid using bran in any form alone and pure, it can be rough and irritating. Use only mixed with other grains, or in its natural state on the grain as it comes.
- Foods must provide abundant minerals and trace minerals. These are normally acquired from mineral rich soils. When soils are depleted of them, they must be replenished. Commercial fertilizers contain only a small number of essential minerals and trace minerals.
- Unless you eat foods grown on total mineral containing soils, it may be necessary to supplement the diet by use of tablets containing the minerals in a concentrated amount.
- Eliminate from the diet, all "empty" foods, mushy foods, refined and commercially processed, prepared; chemically treated, artificially colored, preserved and synthetically prepared foods.

Examples of these types of foods are flaked, puffed, sugared, fancy corn, wheat and rice type cereals, TV dinners, instant foods, quick mixes, candies, puddings, ice cream, etc.

- Don't use more than one concentrated type of protein or starch food at a meal.
- Avoid eating more than one meat meal a day. Meat tends to dry out and harden fecal matter when taken in excess.
- During periods of prolonged fecal retention, avoid intake of table salt. When retained in the body, it can absorb water

from the intestines. Sea salt in water has a beneficial action when constipation is mild.

- Avoid frequent liquid meals, meals low in bulk – consisting mainly of soft, overcooked foods, soups, juices or beverages. These should be taken only in moderation and taken in between meals – not mixed with the solid foods. When taking liquids, they should be spring water and juices.
- Avoid washing down food with liquids. Fluids taken during meals, dilute or flush through the digestive enzymes required for normal digestion. Such a habit always leaves some food poorly digested.
- One tablespoon of any liquid, taken hourly during the day, helps counteract constipation when the stools are hard and dry. It offsets the need for straining. It can soften bowels. It may sound too simple to be effective; however, before resorting to laxatives, try it. Be persistent. It may take up to a month to restore natural, easy eliminations.
- If the stools are too soft and thin or are like diarrhea, and if the bowel movements are less than every two days, keep the fluid intake low. Reverse the suggestions for the dry hard stools. Eat as many dry and bulk foods as possible. Use lots of salads, toasted breads and firm starches.
- During fecal retention, liquids tend to absorb into the body and carry with them toxins and detrimental debris, minerals and gases.

YOUR GALLBLADDER

&

GALLSTONES

Gallbladders are part of our enjoyment to life preservation and restoration of our health. They make many food delicacies available to our bodies.

500,000 gallbladders are removed each year.

Gallbladders are not just spare parts that surgeons like to take out for their profit!

What are gallbladders – what do they do? The gallbladder is a pear-shaped organ and wineskin type pouch. It is located under the liver and stores the bile, which is produced by the liver. It is to the liver as fingers are to the hand. It is a reservoir that stores up to one cup of the three cups of bile that the liver creates in a day. Its role is to contract like a rubber syringe and to force extra amounts of bile into the intestines whenever needed and on a moment's notice.

By its own separate duct, it connects with the bile duct drainage system of the liver.

Through the bile duct, toxic biochemical wastes, toxic materials (copper, zinc, and mercury), drugs and all other liver overloads and excretions are on their way to being eliminated from the body.

Oils (and some fats) are essential to the health of our bodies, as any other food or biochemical. They are our life protectors. They are part of the structures of all our 70 to 100 trillion cells – the cell membranes. They protect those membranes from all toxic or foreign substances or irritants. Without oils, our bodies cannot create hormones. Without hormones, the biochemistry of our bodies would be in chaos. Without oils, our livers could not function and sustain life.

All oils and fats need bile in order to enter into and become a part of the body's functions and health. The greater the intake of fats or oils, the greater is the need for bile. Oils and fats trigger the liver to create and secrete to bile and then to eject this bile into the intestines where it promotes the absorption of the food, oils and fats into the body and activates the intestines to eliminate their toxins and wastes.

Gallbladders are best understood by understanding the function of bile.
Bile is:

- A slightly alkaline syrupy, green liquid. In solution, it contains lecithin, cholesterol, bile pigments and bile salts (manufactured by the liver). Bile drains these out of the liver, via thousands of many ducts that lead to a main duct. A branch of this duct goes to the gallbladder. The gallbladder stores any bile surpluses for extra needs. Bile emulsifies and absorbs all wastes and toxins that have been prepared for elimination by the liver and carries them from the liver to the intestine for their elimination from the body.
- An emulsifier of intestinal contents. Bile emulsification lowers surface tension of the waters in the intestines. This increases the dissolving of water type foods and their mixing with faculty type food substances. This is essential for the body to be able to use them.
- An emulsifier of oils and fats that go into the intestines from the stomach (oils cannot become a part of cells and body functions unless emulsified). The A, D, E, and F vitamin groups are oil soluble and need bile to digest and absorb fats in order to get them into the body and to become involved with the body's physiology.
- A cholesterol carrier: Our brains and organs need cholesterol and the liver is a manufacturer of cholesterol. Bile carries cholesterol from the liver to all parts of our body. The more bile the liver makes, the greater the amount of cholesterol that is available to satisfy the body's needs.
- An inhibitor of excess and abnormal cholesterol production by the liver (the more production of bile), the better the control of the liver production of cholesterol.
- An aid to the digestion of foods, dietary fats attaches themselves to form a coating around foods. This fat coating helps with contact of the digestive enzymes with foods.

Without making contact, the enzyme cannot digest those foods. Food that doesn't digest properly will putrefy or rot. This turns the intestines into a cesspool.

- Bile activates pancreatic secretions. On entering the intestines it sends chemical signals, which triggers the pancreas to secrete its digestive enzymes in exact quantities that is needed for digesting fats and oils.
- A food carrier: bile transports foods through the intestinal wall into the body. Any reduction of the production and excretion of bile by the liver reduces the passage of oils and nutrients through the intestinal wall and into the body.
- A body waste carrier: bile enters the body together with oils. It then combines with used up or toxic body oils, fats and nutrients and returns them to the liver.
- A stool moisturizer and facilitator of BM elimination, bile keeps the intestinal wastes from becoming dry and hard, and difficult to expel.

The forming of gallstones

When oil is lacking in our diet, the gallbladder fails to contract and just starts discharging its reserves of bile. The bile stagnates. If the stagnation is too prolonged, the bile is reabsorbed. Once the liver stops producing bile, the fats in our diet will not be digested since bile emulsifies fats and breaks them down to absorb them. In drying, the bile salts (pigments and calcium that are normally in solution) become concentrated. The bile becomes thick – like molasses in winter. It dries up and turns alkaline.

The increased alkalinity makes the calcium and mineral salts precipitate and form a crystal sediment. This action is just like a high saturation of salt in water as it chills. Mineral salts will remain in solution only if there is enough liquid and acid in the bile to keep them soluble.

The alkalinity of the mineral sediment irritates the inner skin of the gallbladder and causes the gallbladder lining to secrete a thick mucus, whose purpose is to form a film of protection. If the skin that forms the inside wall of the gallbladder is not healthy, excess numbers of its cells dry up and die. They fall off the gallbladder lining and into the thick "syrupy" bile and mucus liquid. This is syrup acts like a glue. It binds the sediment into a stone precipitate.

Too often we introduce into our bodies a second source of a gluing substance – gluten rich foods. Gluten forms a paste, the same as when flour is mixed with water. Our strains of American, Canadian wheat – as a result of making special hybrid forms of wheat – contain five times more gluten than the original wheat strains. Our wheat diet has become a major cause of gallstones. The mixture dries and stones are formed.

Gallstones: Their Nature

There are two types of gallstones: cholesterol stones and bile salt, pigment and calcium stones. Eighty percent of stones are the cholesterol type. Stones vary from grains of sand in size to as big as a small egg. They vary in number from one to hundreds. When gallbladders contract and force out stones larger than the size of the bile duct, they get stuck and block the duct. This is most painful. Blocking the flow of bile from the liver becomes a serious threat to health.

Protecting against Gallstones

The only sure way to prevent stagnation is by eliminating a diet heavy in fats and to activate a contracting and flushing out of bile and stagnating residues by a regular intake of adequate amounts of oils in our diet.

Fats are from animals and cream. Chemically treated commercial oils, (margarine, commercial mayonnaise, salad dressings, spreads, etc.), are the same as fats. (Fats are not oils. Oils are different from fats. Confusing fats with oils come from chemists calling oils fatty acids.) Fats dissolve and store body wastes and toxins. They overload the liver. They interfere with the contraction and secretion of the gallbladder.

Quality oils come in oil rich foods: nuts, seeds, grains, avocados and liver. Oils stimulate the nerves which triggers the muscles of the gallbladder into contracting. They keep livers healthy and functioning at optimum capacity. Oils form coatings around the liver cells, like suits of armor. This coating protects liver cells from the chemicals, toxins, wastes and pollutants that constantly flow through and overload or damage the liver.

Gallbladder Stone "Attacks"

You know you have a gallstone when you experience...

- Steady, severe pain in the area below your right ribs.
- Or pain in the right shoulder or between the shoulder blades.
- Nausea or vomiting.
- Bowel movements that are pale – even yellow or grey. They may have shown this color change for a long time before an attack.
- Pain under and on right side of ribs, halfway between the midline of your body and your side. If the stone is small enough to pass through the gall duct, the pain may last for 20 to 30 minutes. If the stone is large, and cannot pass, the pain may last for hours.

Dissolving and Passing Gallstones

Take lots of quality oils on a regular basis. Take the whole food form oil soluble vitamins: A, D, E, F.

Make sure the body obtains from the diet all the elements required to manufacture lots of good quality bile. This involves a diet well balanced with proteins and minerals, as well as the oils. Diet is discussed in better detail in the book entitled your liver – your laboratory of living.

Use acid solutions that will dissolve the mineral crystals or cholesterols that go into making the stones. Acid acts on the stone surface like sandpaper, peeling off the outer layers. A product called 'D's sodium phosphate' does this very effectively. Bile, in liquid form or capsule, will dissolve out and metabolize minerals and cholesterol.

"Stones cannot form; neither can they stand up under the influence of normal bile." - Dr. J. H. Tilden.

Strengthen the health and integrity of the gallbladder skin lining, mainly with quality oils and Vitamin A – the skin vitamin.

Stop turning your bile into paste. Hold the wheat and the gluten.

To live, eat and drink in ways that impair the liver, and not to eliminate the causes that precipitate minerals which trigger the formation of the stones, is to become prone to a gallstone factory.

Caution: When stones are small enough, the gallbladder after a stimulated normal contraction, will pass them out. As the stone passes through the torturous bile duct, they will scratch the skin lining, making the skin raw and cause pain. These will cause the gall duct to contract and narrow – sometimes too thin to allow passage of even small stones.

Do not ignore excruciating gallstone pain. Seek prompt relief. Pain is an indication that the gall duct has gone into spasm, cramping around and strangling a stone. The use of a strong anti-spasmodic can still make it possible to get the stone to pass through. This would mean medical treatments by your local physician.

To not relieve the pain and spasm would allow the stone to remain lodged in the duct. The pain could go on and on.

Sometimes the following supplements are able to bring about relaxation in the duct and allow the stone to pass through:

i. High zinc enzyme concentrate and beet extract from beets grown in soil that is supersaturated with zinc. Zinc mobilizes more enzyme systems than any other mineral. It activates an increased function of the liver, lowers the very viscosity of bile and increases the drainage through the bile duct. It acts like a liver "Drano". Take six to nine a day during gallstone attacks or if there is nausea, or liver heaviness. Decrease to two to three a day for two to six months to decongest and normalize the liver.
ii. Di-sodium phosphate is a component of bile. It helps to dissolve the crystallized bile salts. Take a half teaspoon in a

glass of warm water before each meal until the stone has dissolved and passed. Take also when constipated.

iii. Betaine hydrochloride, or similar, hydrochloric acid containing supplement. This acid helps dissolve minerals and maintain them in solution.

iv. Take three bile tablets daily to stimulate increased bile flow. Many companies market bile tablets. Cholacol is a brand name of possibly the only commercial form of bile that is detoxified.

v. Go off solid foods and go on a fast for a one to several days. Supersaturate your body with liquids. They help to thin the bile and dissolve mineral crystals.

vi. Take a good quality oil and a glass of fruit juice. This flushes the liver.

It is not only possible for such a program to dissolve stones, but it can be done relatively easy. Sometimes it takes only a few weeks or a few months.

It works much like loading water with salt. It forms a crystal sediment. Heat the water. The crystals dissolve. Chill the water and the salt re-crystallizes. Each time you heat or chill the solution, the same changes take place.

The methods just described...

- Eliminate the causes of the stone formation.
- Reverse the processes of crystallization.
- Dissolve crystals.
- Thin the bile.
- Stimulate the liver and the contractions of the gallbladder.
- Stimulate the flow of bile with its crystals of gravel.

What happens when there is no gallbladder?

Without a gallbladder there is no storehouse or reserve resource to call upon when there is an increased demand for bile, such as after heavy or fatty meals. Your body will no longer be able to completely digest, handle or use the oils and oil rich foods so essential to health.

You may experience no problem other than you must eat conservatively and choose your foods well. You cannot take large amounts of fat or heavy oil meals – not without experiencing discomfort and possibly even liver pain. It is no longer possible to go on binges and celebrate with foods, like rich creams, ice creams, fried foods, chips, pork and fat foods at Christmas, and birthday banquets. Even the leanest of meats contain up to 18 percent fat content. This can be too much for a body with the absence of a gallbladder.

If a problem arises at any time, you will probably need to take extra amounts of bile in tablet form. When you live without a gallbladder, it is advisable at all times to keep some bile supplements on hand. You may need them.

If you want to live with your smile, be most careful of your bile.

YOUR LIVER:
Laboratory for Living

To understand your liver, its nature, its functions, its wisdom, is to master the most valuable and essential information about health and healing and prevention of disease.

Your liver is your life.

If one were to attempt to build a laboratory that would perform all of the functions of a simple five-pound liver, it would have to be the size of a small city, and operate by the personnel equal to the population of that city.

The liver, its marvels and miracles, is one of the best-kept secrets of the healing professions. Our livers are the laboratories of almost everything in our living. It is the greatest of all living organs. No other organ plays such an enormous role in health and healing. Perfect livers prevent, cure or are necessary agents of curing of all diseases. No chronic or degenerative type of disease can exist for any length of time when livers perfectly function.

A healthy liver can withstand the worst onslaughts and abuses we can impose upon it. It can suffer excesses and overloads for many years before its reserves are depleted and before experiencing noticeable distress signs or symptoms. The liver's quietude is misleading. It induces us to believe that our livers are quite healthy and leaves us with a false sense of security; hence, we neglect caring for our livers.

However, it is not possible for our livers to be neglected, exposed to and affected by all the daily stresses, abnormalities and ecological hazards of our civilization, and remain healthy. Our general health, our resistance to disease, our abilities to live and enjoy life parallels the condition of our livers.

According to *Worldwide Abstracts of General Medicine*, liver disease is probably the most serious chronic illness facing the world today. Over 25 million people in America have some serious liver ailment. Over 50,000 Americans die of liver disease each year. It is the third leading cause of death for people between the ages of 25 to 59.

Everybody owes it to themselves to become acquainted with and make friends with their liver, especially those with a health problem. To not be familiar with the world of your liver is to be deprived of knowing that a perfectly functioning liver is the key to the assurance of and the means of maintaining or restoring perfect health.

Health starts in, and is created, balanced, maintained and protected by our livers.

When there is illness and that illness persists for any length of time, it should be obvious that the body's ability to protect itself from disease has been lost – some of the healing properties are not performing as they could and should be. Something needs help.

In the course of searching for a way or a system to restore wellbeing to an ailing body, logic enjoins us to find out how our body heals – which organs, biochemical systems and healing agents reinstate healing? What can be done to mobilize all agents and restore all processes to their peak healing ability again?

A trend in healing professions is to treat our body's obvious needs and symptoms, and unfortunately, too often only those. Medical doctors generally don't examine or pay close attention to livers or their inadequacies. Not unless there is a serious liver disease. They have been trained to disregard livers. They treat only organs or tissues that are diseased or symptoms that relate to them. They pay little attention to the liver's importance to heal those organs, tissues or diseases. They are trained to use drugs and chemicals as the best and only remedies for controlling diseases.

Limiting medical training and therapies to the use of drugs creates monstrous health and healing problems. Every drug, every chemical, every abnormal substance is a liver hazard – a liver poison. Every drug and chemical damages the liver. They destroy the enzymes which are the agents of all liver healing and of all liver function. No drug should be prescribed during an illness (except in life-threatening emergencies, of course), for every drug hampers the organ and processes that cure illness.

In order to continue prescribing drugs, doctors are conditioned to block considerations of the liver from their minds. Medical therapy is controlled by the drug companies. Either prescribe drugs or lose your license. Not to prescribed drugs would put the drug companies out of business. This is not allowable. Much about the world of the liver must remain a medical obscurity.

The result of this lack of consideration for the supreme importance of the liver is that little good, clear, simple, practical and comprehensive information about it is available. Even to doctors.

Even holistic oriented doctors often just treat the negatives that manifest as disease. They may correct general body deficiencies, toxicities and give counsel for the mind, emotions and lifestyle. They may provide the best possible tools for healing. However, too often insufficient consideration is given to what is in our body and in its healing processes to use those tools. Inadequate support is often rarely provided to the healing organ that has to do all the work.

Healing, in a way, can be compared to building or repairing a house. All the materials required for completing the job are of little value without a top rate carpenter to make fashion and shape them. That carpenter has to be in excellent health and well nourished. Our body's builder and repair expert is our liver.

Libraries of information about liver biochemistry do exist. It is there, it is available. Herbs for the liver, folklore remedies, homeopathic remedies and liver acupuncture points, have been known and used effectively for centuries in many parts of the world. Medical research has discovered and revealed the nature of cells and of enzymes which are the agents of all cell functions and healing. Unfortunately, too little of medical research findings reached the desks of doctors or the disease needs of patients.

The liver is the largest internal body organ. It performs more functions than any other organ. It is the major organ for:

- The detoxification, neutralization and elimination of all body wastes and toxins.
- Storing glycogen, which when in need, the adrenal gland hormones transfer and release into the body for needed usable sugar and energy.
- Storing iron in healthy, utilizable form.
- Performing almost all the functions of healing and protection against disease.

- Manufacturing bile which emulsifies and makes absorbable the oils and the oil soluble vitamins so essential to health. Bile also activates toxins and elimination by the intestines and creates the alkaline reaction, which is the essential healthy biochemical intestinal environment – the milieu which prevents putrefaction.
- There is no adequate or normal flushing out of intestinal toxins, poisons, drugs and/or body wastes without the activity of the liver and its bile.

The liver will be considered in these aspects:

- What is the liver?
- What are its marvels?
- The myriad functions of the liver.
- Your liver and your immunity.
- Your liver and your detoxification.

The factors essential for normal liver...

- Enzymes
- Oils
- Proteins
- Vitamins and carbohydrates

Various liver ailments:

- Causes of liver illnesses and problems
- Liver restoration and maintenance
- Diet and nutrition
- Lifestyles, emotions, exercise and the liver
- Some “don’ts” of liver care
- Detoxifying your liver
- Special cautions and counsels
- Summary

Most of us take our livers for granted. If you have done this, it would do you well to check the following symptoms and discomforts. They can indicate possible liver weakness, toxicities and or deficiencies – even if there is no liver disease.

- Sluggishness experienced when rising in the morning.
- For the first hour or two, to get active and going requires effort, pushing self, an act of one's will.
- Energies and vitality reserves are low. Feeling low, down, negative, sickly and even depressed.
- Ambitions and enthusiasms aren't as they used to be.
- Decision making is difficult and may require a real effort.
- You are not optimistic, happy as you used to be.
- Declining physical strength and endurance.
- Occasional experiences of nausea, especially in the mornings. Feelings of heaviness, or pressure (like lead) in your head.
- Heaviness, fullness or discomfort feeling under the right ribs. This discomfort is worst when bending over.
- Breathing difficulties experienced when climbing stairs.
- Shallow complexion of the skin, with considerable itching.
- Appetite not as good as it used to be.
- Appetite is poor, especially in the hours just after rising.
- Blue "spider web" lines (veins) visible in cheeks, nose, upper or lower chest or lower abdomen.
- Sex urges are not what they used to be.
- Slow, sluggish bowel movements.
- The bowel movement color is occasionally or frequently lighter than dark brown, even orange or grey.
- You often pass intestinal gas.
- Your blood cholesterol readings are high.
- You have an illness that refuses to heal.

Or one or more of the diseases below, caused by the impurities of blood that did not get properly filtered and purified by the liver, which pass into the head and brain.

Faulty concentration, creativity problems, insomnia, depression, mental debility, mental senility, losses of memory, imagination problems.

Abnormalities that create liver symptoms

We, and the conditions we live in, subject our livers to more insults, injuries, stresses and hazards than we do to any other organ. No liver can continuously, and for years, handle all the overloads of body toxins and waste listed below:

- Cigarettes and alcohol
- Junk, synthetic, counterfeit and artificial foods
- Fat, fried foods, sugar excesses
- Three thousand toxic chemicals, food additives and preservatives (food embalming chemicals) in our foods protein molecules of undigested foods
- Chemicals, pesticides and fertilizers
- Chlorine and fluoride in our water
- Fumes of natural gas and air-conditioners
- Foods destroyed by microwaves, overcooking, cooking in aluminum, pressure cooking, canning and freezing
- Pollutants of air and industry traffic
- Various radiations that's super saturate our environment
- Emotional traumas
- Negative attitudes and stresses, even noises

The forces of health battle endlessly in our livers for supremacy against the negative and destructive forces, toxins, overloads, excesses, lifestyle abuses and abnormalities of our civilized living. All the body garbage overloads and plugs up livers. Livers become saturated like sponges in a dirty sink. This is liver congestion.

Our excesses, habits and lifestyle affect the liver's ability to function just as much, and often more, than to the foods, drugs, pollutants, alcohol, and other hazards. Yet, when damaged or diseased, livers literally have unique abilities to constantly and repeatedly regenerate itself many times over.

Your Liver in Perspective

Your liver is a four-to-five pound organ situated mostly on the right side of the body, under your diaphragm and almost hidden under and protected by your ribs. It is next to the skin, the body's largest organ.

Livers are made up of approximately 300 billion cells. These cells are grouped in special functional units call lobules. Each lobule is made up of approximately 350,000 cells of several different kinds. Lobules are organized into microscopic filters – each about the size of a pinhead. Each filter intercepts and purifies blood coming in from every cell and organ.

The highly magnified pinhead-sized liver lobules are responsible for many thousands more biochemical reactions and chores than any other tissue.

Approximately five cups of blood pass through the liver every minute – about 1200 pints of blood in 24 hours. Blood passes into the liver through the portal vein. Purified and refilled with nutrients, the blood is then pumped by the heart to the lungs for oxygen.

There are two blood vessel systems – two sources of blood flow to the liver. One brings in food molecule from the stomach and intestinal lines. The liver converts these into nutrients that can be used up by cells. The other major vein brings in blood from the whole body, as well as from the lymphatic system. This blood is for filtering and detoxifying.

Impurities, wastes, toxins and abnormal substances that pour into the liver come from all our tissues. They are microscopic sewer pipes that drain the cell wastes, created by their activities (metabolism). These drainage pipes are called lymph channels. Microscopic channels join together to form larger channels, then major channels, then a main channel which dumps into the bloodstream, just above the heart. The blood carries the toxins to the liver for processing. The lymphatic system is a network of vessels as abundant and complex as the overall blood circulation.

Interference with the flow of the blood through the liver, affects the liver as it does the whole body. (Other factors also interfere with the blood flow: poor pumping of a tired, diseased, or nutrient-starved heart muscle, blood that is too thick, blood clots clogging up the arteries and tumors pressing on the blood vessels.)

The Marvels and Functions of the Liver

Performing the greatest number of functions of the whole body, the liver is the most hearty, versatile and amazing of all organs. Our livers possess almost infinite abilities, functions and endurance. These include powers to heal, normalize and balance any body's abnormality and disease.

To duplicate the thousands of biochemical functions of a simple five-pound liver would require a laboratory the size of a large city, complete with equipment, technicians and personnel.

- **Livers are enzyme creating and enzyme storing organs.**

To understand our livers, we need to understand enzymes. Enzymes are the agents that make possible the function of every organ in the body and of every process of living.

Our livers manufacture thousands of different types of valuable and powerful enzymes. These liver enzymes transform substances that are brought to the liver from the intestines, into whatever nutrients are needed by every cell in our body. Livers chemically process and counteract all abnormal substances, wastes, debris of dying cells, worn out tissues, the chemical refuse, fumes and garbage that all organs of the body generate in their functions of living, the pollutants from food, water and air, and from our environment.

They are; however, not able to overcome all the side effects and poisons of medical drugs, pesticides, radiations, chemicals and poisons from modern industry.

- **Livers create vigor, vitality, energy and cells**

Liver enzymes, by splitting food molecules into ways similar to what happens in an atom bomb, create our life and life force.

The liver enzymes continue to transform food into materials for building cells. Liver cells absorb and store carbohydrates in a special chemical form called glycogen. When our bodies require more fuel in order to perform all its functions, the liver converts the glycogen molecules into readily available sugars and energy.

- **Livers create energies and fuels for our muscles**

Muscles depend on the liver for their strength and efficiency, and for the fuel foods they use in their efforts. Liver enzymes process starch, sugar, carbohydrates, oils and fats.

The liver salvages toxic waste products (lactic acid) from excess muscle activity and transforms them back into glycogen. When extra energy is required to handle extra activities and stresses, a hormone from the adrenal gland (adrenalin) activates the release of glycogen so that it can flow back into the body.

- **Livers are nutrient stockpilers and "warehouses". Livers are storehouses for, and provide when needed...**

Proteins and amino acids required and used for healing, restoring, repairing and maintaining integrity, and functions of the body.

- All proteins must be in molecular food forms that can be transformed into body and liver cells. Only when natural, unprocessed, not overcooked, nor chemically treated, hydrolysed, liquefied or in the form of isolated amino acids can proteins be used, stored or transformed into body and liver cells.

- Oils, sugars, enzymes, cholesterol and thousands of biochemical.
- Minerals, primarily iron, zinc, copper, manganese and phosphorus.

  Livers provide, regulate and control the vitamins and minerals essential to the creation of blood in the marrow of our bones, namely the A, B, B12, D and K groups.

- **Livers create immunity-resistance against disease. They:**

  - Heal, repair, restore and rebuild cells.
  - Normalize and control body biochemical and all substances and nutrients which create our bodies.
  - Stabilize a body, mind and emotional balance.
  - Detoxify and eliminate toxins.
  - Protect, defend, resist and immunize against diseases.

With a perfectly functioning liver, no one would be a slave to any disease beyond a very short time. There would not be any serious health breakdown or degenerative disease, including cancer, AIDS, ulcers, multiple sclerosis, arthritis, heart disease, neurasthenia, mental and emotional disturbances, kidney, lung, skin and other diseases.

Liver enzymes protect cells and protect them from the damaging effects of chemicals and pollutants.

- **Livers create and secrete an anti-histamine (Yakitron)**

The liver produces natural antihistamines and provide the same relief against allergies and toxins as those manufactured by drug companies, without any undesirable side effects.

Histamine molecules are in every cell. When cells die and disintegrate, they release these molecules into the surrounding fluids. This histamine is an irritant which, in making contact with a nearby cell, whips it, multiply and divide. By this means, cells that die are immediately and automatically placed by new, young and strong cells. Histamine excesses are toxic. They create symptoms and distresses, which we know as allergies.

Histamine is also a factor in the multiplication of cells in cancer, as these grow into and become tumors. Poisons or carcinogens that create cancer, cause greater numbers of cells to die than when the body is healthy. The death of so many cells at one time releases excesses of histamine.

- **Livers transform byproducts of faulty protein digestion (ammonia) into urea.**

Kidneys cannot dispose the high amounts of byproducts of food and cell degradation without the intervention of the liver.

- **Livers manufacture substances that cause the blood to clot (Vitamin K and others).**

In doing so, they stop bleeding and hemorrhaging, even bleeding to death.

- **Livers manufacture anticoagulants called heparin.**

Heparin prevents the formation of clots and thrombi. If anti-coagulants were lacking, blood would readily clot. The clots would block arteries. They could cause a fatal heart attack or stroke.

- **Livers neutralize, inactivate and balance sex hormones whenever these hormones are in excess.**

- **Livers protect and stabilize our minds and nerves.**

By maintaining balance of all body biochemical, and eliminating all their excesses; maintain normalness, quickness, sharpness and agilities of our mental abilities.

- **Liver enzymes digest and disintegrate worn-out blood and white blood cells.**

They recycle whatever cell elements that can be used or are needed by the body. They reject and eliminate those that cannot be used.

- **Livers play a major role in control of blood pressures.**

The heart constantly pumps blood. A congested liver blocks the blood's return from every part of the body back to the heart. The volume of blocked blood gradually overfills the veins and arteries. The pressure in the blocked circulation has to rise. An answer is of course to flesh out, clean out and decongest the liver.

- **Liver enzymes destroy viruses, bacteria and bacterial poisons and flush them out of the body.**

- **Livers are master body detoxifiers.**

Livers are our shock troops, our frontline defenders against all health hazards. They neutralize, detoxifies, render harmless and rid our bodies of all their wastes, dying cell debris, poisons, pollutants, chemical drugs and all the substances that our bodies cannot use.

Liver enzymes detoxify by combining molecules of minerals and carbohydrates with the toxic substances, which previously separated from nutrients and other body substances. In this way the liver handles and gets rid of about 40 percent of all harmful substances in our body.

Possibly the body's most effective detoxifying liver substance is one called "glucuronic acid". This acid is synthesized in the liver by the aid of Vitamin C from glycogen, sugar and lactic acid.

When one's liver is unable to handle toxic overloads, it pass these on to other organs of detoxification and elimination. The first overload-handling organ is the kidney.

- **Livers are toxin and waste eliminators.**

Livers manufacture bile. They use bile as a solvent to absorb the poisons. Bile carries the poisons through the bile ducts into the intestines to be eliminated from the body.

Bile: Its Functions and Actions

- Bile is the most important agent of digestion. The bile in our intestines emulsifies the oils and fats of foods we digest, including the oil soluble vitamins. This emulsification makes possible the absorption of essential nutrients.
- Bile is essential for detoxification and elimination. It is a major stimulant of bowel movements. The bile and its toxins instigate the contractions of the intestinal muscles by irritating the intestinal walls. This, in turn, forces the excretion of fecal matter.
- Problems of elimination are often the effects of a sluggish, under functioning liver that does not manufacture enough bile. Without bile, carrying off toxins and wastes to the intestines is reduced. Flushing out waste and toxins from the colon slows down. Stagnating toxins build up.
- Our bodies poorly tolerate stagnating fecal matter. Toxins and poisons that are not flushed out, filter through the intestinal wall. They re-absorbed back into the blood and tissues. The blood vessels carry the impurities back into the liver. The latter creates liver trouble.
- Bile plays a major role in the control of obesity. It dissolves fat stored in the fatty tissues and help carry it to the liver for processing, then to the intestines for elimination.
- Normal bile levels decrease appetite and hunger. Its use as a therapy is too frequently disregarded.
- Bile is a solvent which absorbs cholesterol and carries it, by means of the blood stream, to every tissue of the body. Cell membranes cannot be strong, healthy or function normally without normal, healthy cholesterol.

- Bile dissolves and carries out of the intestines all abnormal toxic cholesterol.
- Bile is a chemical messenger which, on reaching the intestines, signals the pancreas to create and secrete its fat-digesting enzymes (both of food and body fat) called lipase.
- Bile is an emulsifier, which helps substances insoluble in water, mix with those that are water-soluble.

Assessing bile levels and sufficiency

Normal, adequate amounts of bile are determined by their action on fecal matter and bowel movements. Bile creates the dark brown color of the bowel movements. It keeps the stool soft and easy to eliminate. When the stools are pale brown, orange, yellow or grey, and or when they are dry and hard, and need forcing, and take a long time to pass, the bile secretion of the liver is too low.

All the thousands of biochemical transformations that take place in the liver make it the laboratory of living, the most active, the most powerful organ of our living. Everything that is unnatural, dead and in disharmony with the nature of our bodies, can be a hazard to the optimal health and functioning of our livers, and to its health in general. Our health cannot continually survive the biochemically denatured, polluted, conditions of our Western civilization. When the liver no longer functions as it should, almost every other part and function of our body and mind will also be affected. To retain optimal wellbeing and healthy livers, we must have to live close to nature (ideally on a tropical island) free of stress, living true to our individual natures and purposes of life – completely fulfilling our potentials and our abilities. We would have to eat by picking our foods from trees or from their original plants and not allowed artificial, synthetic, chemically treated, de-vitalized or denatured foods created by the genius of so-called scientific minds. Our lives would have to be free of all the negativities and atrocities we perpetrate on ourselves.

Livers are vulnerable. They can be victims of common hazards. When we destroy nature – our nature – we destroy our livers too.

Factors that hamper liver functions

The following lists hazards in order of their importance and abilities to damage the liver...

- Emotional traumas, stresses and grief.
- Negative emotions: hatred, anger, fears and anxieties.
- Drugs, prescription drugs, chemicals, poisons and pesticides.
- Non-foods, counterfeit foods, dead foods, junk, instant, stale, overcooked, microwaved foods and sweet foods.
- Inadequately digested or unusable foods.
- Body pollutants, wastes, cell debris, toxins, abnormal and foreign substances, and allergens.
- Regular, excess alcohol and soft drink consumption.
- Environmental pollutants and radiations.
- The stagnation and accumulation and failure to eliminate the body pollutants.
- Chemical additives, colorings, flavorings, fluorides and chlorines; air and water pollutions.

All the above hazards affect more than just our livers. Each organ functions closely with every other organ and every other energy system of our body. When the life force of the liver is in plenty supply and flowing freely, all other organs will be well nourished and functioning as they should. When there are liver problems, there are problems, or early stages of problems in every organ and tissue of the body.

The organ that first and possibly most affects the liver is the pancreas.

Inadequate or Secretion of Pancreatic Enzymes

Pancreatic enzymes complete the breakdown of proteins into amino acids. They process oil and sugar foods into usable molecules. A failure of the pancreas to produce its full quota of digestive enzymes at every meal will produce incomplete digested foods. Each small fraction of the daily intake of food that escapes being processed by the pancreatic enzymes, rots or putrefies and creates intestinal gas.

Sugar or starch-type foods ferment and protein type foods putrefy. The end products of rotting and putrefaction are very toxic. Intestinal gas is almost as toxic as small doses of arsenic. This poison paralyzes the intestinal muscles and blocks their contractions and elimination of fecal matter. Fecal matter then stagnates in the bowels.

Intestinal gases ferment and putrefaction fills the intestines. They stretch the intestinal walls like a balloon. This stretching separates cells and creates millions of microscopic openings – like pinhole size windows. Through these openings, like escape valves, the intestinal toxins and gases filter into the body. Some will pass into the blood. The blood carries them to the liver and brain. Intestinal gas is an important part of the body and liver toxicity.

To protect our livers and our lives, all undigested foods, food overloads, every substance that is abnormal, dead or irritating, as well as everything that hampers digestion, stresses and tensions, and allergies must be eliminated from our bodies.

Emotional Trauma, Shocks, Stresses

The organ that relates most closely with our emotional states is the liver. Severe emotional trauma undermines and exhausts the liver the most, more than months of alcohol excesses. The emotion closely related to a disturbed liver is anger. We are more prone to anger when our livers are congested, sluggish and slow, and under functioning. Anger weakens both the body's energies and the detoxifying functions of the liver.

Depressed livers leave mind and emotional depressions. Fears, worries, anxieties overwork and drain liver resources.
Therapies that restore and support the liver greatly benefit states of mental and emotional anguish.

Drugs, Chemicals, Poisons and Pollutants

All drugs, including prescription medications, antibiotics, sedatives, chemical hormones, pleasure drugs, and chemotherapy, etc., destroy enzymes and damage livers. All chemicals force the liver to mobilize enzymes to neutralize breakdown and render poisons harmless. All chemicals and drugs destroy and deplete liver enzymes.

Drugs are specifically contraindicated when livers are congested and their functions depressed (except in emergencies). Taking a single drug can block or inhibit liver restoration, its functions and healing abilities. Synthetic and (so-called) "natural" vitamins, minerals and/or amino acids when refined and processed, and devoid of their enzymes produce similar effects on the liver as do drugs.

Our bodies can only use substances which are alive and in which all enzymes, minerals, trace minerals and proteins, required to nourish, protect and heal our bodies are present.

Radiation

Radiation is the most destructive of all forces. It devastates and destroys enzymes and the chromosomes which produce those enzymes. Current world atmospheric radiation levels are approximately triple our body tolerance.

Allergens

All foods are substances, to which a body is allergic to, acts the same as drugs, toxins or chemicals. They require and burn up greater amount of enzymes than do substances which the body can readily metabolize. One cup of coffee, one cigarette, one serving of wheat or sugar to which one is allergic has 10 times more toxic effects on our body than the same items when well handled by the body's processes.

Stagnating body wastes, cell debris and toxins; toxins retained in our bodies by constipation

Amounts equivalent to the quantities of substances ingested each day must also be eliminated. For every substantial meal there *must* be one bowel movement. If not, the retained surpluses filter through our tissues and exert harmful effects.

Lack of sleep, rest, or relaxation

Most of the nutrient and toxin processing required to replenish and regenerate the whole body takes place only when sleeping and resting. Too few hours of these deprive the liver of the time it requires to complete the work of breaking down and eliminating poisons, and creating the nutrients required for cell growth and repair.

Overcooking Foods

Excess heat destroys and renders useless and inassimilable, up to 95 percent of proteins. Heating foods above 165°F or 70°C destroys enzymes. The higher the heat, the more enzymes are destroyed. Overcooking food is like baking clay in an oven. The clay becomes so hard it can no longer be molded into pottery. The food undergoes changes, which makes is impossible for the body to use.

Cooking Proteins

Cooking promotes the release of protein molecules of the original meat or food before the digestive processes have the chance to transform them into harmless and also readily usable amino acid molecules. These foreign protein molecules have a different chemical nature and structure than those of the human body. Abnormal proteins are highly toxic. Researchers who have only injected isolated proteins into the bloodstream of an animal, observed that they were capable of killing the animal. If absorbed into the bloodstream of humans, a severe allergic reaction will happen, which will result in severe shock.

Overindulgences: Dietary Excesses

The excess intakes of wrong foods, dead foods, junk foods, synthetic foods, chemically treated and overcooked foods. Over eating overloads the livers and overloading is liver fatigue. Food excesses (even quality foods) increase the amounts of enzymes needed to metabolize them. They deplete liver enzyme reserves.

Foodless, Counterfeit, Refined, Processed and Non-foods

Livers cannot remain healthy, if not nourished with live, natural, total, enzyme-rich foods. Nor can it transform dead, "foodless" foods into molecules needed and utilizable by body cells. All foods and substances that are not as natural as in their original state, such as growing plants, or that are stale, chemically treated, radiated, processed and refined, canned, treated with preservatives and additives are hazardous to livers.

All dead, refined, processed, junk foods, those from which the natural content of vitamins, minerals, enzymes and/or life forces have either been eliminated by commercial extraction and processing, or have been destroyed by heat, oxygen, chemicals or radiation, combined with, worn out and burned up enzymes. They deplete reasonable reserves of body enzymes the same as do drugs, chemicals and poisons.

Foods to Avoid...

All synthetic foods:

TV dinners, Nutrisweet, Aspartame, artificial sweeteners and cream substitute coffee mixes (every ingredient of Coffeemate is a chemical or drug).

Canadian/American wheat, white flour and flour products

Man-made strains of wheat contain five times more gluten than nature's original strains. The same as making glue by combining flour and water, gluten makes our blood excessively thick. Thickened blood creates serious circulation problems. Excesses of wheat gluten can congest and plug up a liver.

All Commercial Boxed, Dry, (sweetened) Cereals, such as:

Cornflakes, Shredded Wheat, Total, All Bran and all the variations of such cereals. Research tests have shown that animals eating the cardboard used to box the cereals survive longer than those animals that ate the cereal foods.

All Rich, High-fat-containing Foods

Fats make livers sluggish. They slow down or block the flushing out of liver toxins by its bile.

All Sweets, Sugars and Sugar-rich Foods

Desserts, diet foods, cookies, white sugar, ice creams, candies, chocolate bars, jams, jellies and syrups. One can get too much of even the quality sugars, such as honey and the sugars in fruits, especially in juice form. The maximum body daily tolerance of sugars from any source is four ounces. Up to two- to-three tablespoons a day of pasteurized honey is acceptable and very beneficial to livers.

It is most important to avoid high sugar/starch breakfasts, such as restricting the first food intake of the day to coffee with toast, buns or bagels, or to only fruits and fruit juices. Sugars from such foods absorb rapidly into the blood. Rapid absorption pushes blood sugar levels too high. The pancreas is forced to secrete large amounts of insulin to balance these sugar levels. The insulin burns up the excess sugars. It does this in a very short time. The insulin lasts for up to 40 hours and continues to burn sugars that are supposed to be maintained in reserve in our bodies, livers and blood. Our blood sugar levels continue to drop until we experience loss of energy, fatigue, exhaustion, listlessness, dullness, poor concentration – even headaches. This is hypoglycemia.

Our liver sugar levels also drop. The liver cannot function with without large amounts of sugar. Its thousands of essential body functions slow down.

Brain sugar levels also drop. The brain needs and use as much sugar as does the whole body. The brain and mind abilities drop.

All sort all soft drinks, sodas, synthetic, chemical, counterfeit, artificial fruit juices and juices made from "crystals".

All rancid, old, stale, chemically treated commercial oils.

All grocery store salad dressings, mayonnaises, stale, rancid, hydrogenated oils, margarines, peanut butters, spreads, all non-vacuum packed wheat germs, and its oils.

All High-fat Foods

Pork, ham, bacon, lard, Crisco, shortening, French fries, chips and all fried foods.

Don't use fats or oils in combination with high starch, sweets and sugar foods. These adhere to and coat the outer surfaces of foods. This coating makes it impossible for the stomach and the pancreatic enzymes to make contact with the food substances and digest them. The undigested foods then rot or putrefy in the gut.

All Shelled, Stale, Rancid, Salted, Roasted Peanuts

All artificially preserved, colored foods, food additives, modifiers, food chemicals, food coloring, flavorings, thickeners and preservatives

There is no such thing as a preservative. To preserve is to mummify. So call "preservatives" are "embalming fluids". To mummify is to destroy the life force and the enzymes of foods.
The most destructive form of food preserving is radiation. It destroys as much in foods as it does in the human body.

All Smoked Meats, Fish and Foods

The "smoke" flavor is now artificially produced by chemicals.

All canned foods, vegetables, fishes, meats, especially canned tuna and salmon.

Frozen foods:

Except for frozen beans and seed foods (corn, peas, beans) use only fresh vegetables whenever they are in season.

All Re-heated, Stored Foods

The longer they are stored, the more dead and less nutritious they are.

All Overcooked, Microwave or Pressure-cooked foods

All these methods destroy food enzymes and render the foods almost unusable.

Powerful microwaves physically shatter protein molecules. Shattering denatures proteins. They are no longer able to assimilate. The body cannot use them. Denatured proteins are toxic. They reduce immunity and resistance to disease; they contribute to cancer and degenerations.

All processed protein foods: bologna, wieners, salami, canned meats, etc. These too are denatured and toxic.

Carefully choose foods in the ways you combine them. Don't eat/mix at the same meals foods that are:

Left column foods mixes poorly with the right column foods.

ACID		ALKALINES
Highly concentrated starch, refined sweets, sugar foods, fruit juices	NOT WITH	High concentrate, overcooked, processed, proteins
Oils, creams, fats, oil rich foods	NOT WITH	The proteins above, starches, sweets, sugars, fruits

Foods, when mixed with or in contact with other foods, react together as do other chemicals. Acid foods react with alkaline foods. The reaction changes the nature of both.

They denature each other. They become non-foods, poorly unusable by the body. This can apply even to some equality foods of different acid/alkaline natures when mixed together.

This counsel concerns mostly the concentrated foods, such as high concentrated proteins (meats, beans, millet), sugars, foods rich in these and the high concentrated sugars of fruit juices and fats, and oils - not the quality oil-rich foods, such as grains, seeds, nuts, fresh from shells.

It is not chemically reasonable to mix in the stomach two or more foods of opposite acid/alkaline natures at the same time. The stomach needs to secrete generous amounts of its hydrochloric acid to digest the alkaline foods and only sparse amounts for foods which are already acid.

Vegetables, fish and meats are alkaline in nature. Fruits, grains, seeds, nuts, sugars, sweets are all acids.

Some foods are to be used in moderation:

- **Starches, high gluten foods, breads**: Breads are overcooked, highly concentrated starches.
- **Fresh meats:** Preferably use wild game meats, lean meats, fowl and chicken when and if they are healthy and organic. Better is the flesh meats from healthy liver, healthy animals.
- **Eggs:** Healthy eggs are quite acceptable. They do not increase blood cholesterol levels. They contain lecithin, which will lower abnormal cholesterol excesses.

To be healthy, the eggs must...

- Be from healthy, grain-fed chickens
- Be fertilized
- Be only lightly and slowly cooked – never hard
- Never fried or hard-boiled

Large quantities of fruit at any one meal, as discussed above.

Citrus fruits, and especially their juices, taken in excess, the citric acid (in citrus fruits) binds itself to calcium. It turns calcium into insoluble and unusable calcium salts or crystals. These crystals can deposit in joints and cause pain and arthritis. Citrus foods are from tropical climates and are desirable during tropical-type warm weather seasons to replace minerals lost through the skin when abundantly perspiring.

Alcohol, alcohol beverages, mixes, soft drinks

As harmful as alcohol is to livers, it is neither the only nor the most serious cause of liver ailments. However, more chemicals, flavorings, colorings, preservatives, additives are used in the preparation of commercial cheaper wines, beers and liquors that are used in most foods. These have a far greater toxic effect on livers than does the alcohol itself. All of these force the liver to use and burn up large amounts of enzymes, especially of the vitamin B complex group.

All the above eventually tax livers beyond their capacities and reserves. Livers break down under constant and extreme overloads. They lose their battle against endless mistreatments, abuses and neglect. Owners of weak livers lose their health-maintaining and regenerating powers. As long as livers are in excellent condition, there is no serious or degenerative disease that could survive longer than days or weeks. As livers fail, so does health and the resistance to almost any disease.

Diseases arising from liver problems

Inadequately functioning livers give rise to the following symptoms and diseases:

- Breakdown of immunity – host resistance
- Exhaustion, fatigue and burnouts
- High blood pressure

All blood must pass through the liver, as it is being pumped through to the heart. The swollen tissues of the congested liver hinder this blood flow. The heart continues to pump blood into the liver. When blood can't get through, its volume accumulates in the blood vessels throughout the body. This creates an increase of pressure against the blood vessel walls. The result is an increase in blood pressure.

Thrombosis

When blood is hampered from flowing through the liver, because of liver tissue congestion and swelling, it stagnates. Stagnating blood tends to form clots.

Fatty Livers

In normal livers, fats are not a problem. Liver enzymes, vitamins, especially choline and bile normally dissolve fats and flush them out of the liver. When fats are ingested in excess, there is an absence of these fat metabolizers, and when the blood cannot pass freely through the liver, fat molecules accumulate and form deposits. The liver becomes a storage bin for fats, food excesses, harmful wastes, toxins and blood and body poisons. Abnormal foods and chemicals in our diets, body toxins, tobacco, drugs, arsenic, phosphorous, alcohol and pollutants seriously aggravate this condition.

Cirrhosis of the liver

Cirrhosis is a state of liver degeneration where fat cells replace a number of the liver cells as they die or degenerate from a lack of proper nutrition and care, and from the effects of toxins, drug overloads and poisons. When contact with the poisons is prolonged, or the poisons are excessive, cirrhosis and death can result.

Cirrhosis is acclaimed by the medical profession as incurable. It is incurable if only drugs are used as therapies. However, normalizing all the liver requirements with health-restoring regimes, diets and therapies, and if the condition is not too advanced or in extreme, it is possible, over a period of years, for the liver to grow back to normal.

Psoriasis, eczema, acne, skin rashes or other skin diseases

Healthy oils protect skin against skin diseases. Abnormal toxic fats and oils, and those which are not thoroughly digested by pancreatic enzymes and not properly handled by the liver; not solubilized by choline and bile, will form fat deposits in skin. They become skin irritants and toxins, and create diseased skin conditions.

Kidney Diseases

The liver transforms nitrogen into urea. Our kidneys cannot dispose the waste without this prior processing of nitrogen wastes by the liver. When excess toxins and wastes from the liver exhausts the kidney, kidney diseases results.

Pneumonia and Lung Diseases

These two are very much liver dependent and related to the health of the liver. When kidneys are no longer able to handle the overload of toxins dumped onto them by the liver, they in turn, pass some of the overloads onto the lungs. Overloads that become too much for the lungs will then buildup and stagnate in lung tissues. They irritate the lung tissues and cause them to secrete mucus as a means of coating and protecting the lung linings from these irritants. The combination of toxins and mucus start to fill the lungs and create the condition known as pneumonia.

Hemorrhoids

Hemorrhoids are not really a disease, they are a symptom – a red flag that the body uses as an SOS – a danger signal, indicating that the liver is overloaded and swollen. They can also be caused by pregnancy, tumors or constipation.

Blood that cannot flow through a seriously congested liver will back up in the veins going to the liver. Those veins will swell up due to an increased volume created by the flow slow down. Swelling will occur throughout the abdominal veins right down to those in the walls of the rectum. The rectal veins are some of the thinnest and most fragile. It takes very little pressure to make them crack or break and allow blood to leak out. Nature intended these rectal veins to be fragile. Their swelling and breaking, often followed by bleeding, is our body's way of making us aware of restrictions impeding the flow of blood.

Hemorrhoids are a safety valve. If the pressure should ever build up to a point where it would break the veins, nature prevents this from becoming an internal hemorrhage by letting the blood escape to the outside, through the rectum instead of the abdominal cavity where it would do serious harm.

The symptom of rectal itching is an added body signal. Itching is our body's way of telling us that the tissues in the itchy area are not getting the nutrients and oxygen they need. Itching makes us want to scratch; scratching forces more blood back into the starved tissues.

Hemorrhoids are prompts telling us to look after our livers

Hemorrhoid veins should not be surgically removed. This also removes their value as warning signals against impending high blood pressure or liver congestion. Instead of surgery, treat hammered hemorrhoids by decongesting the liver or by ridding the body of any other obstruction or pressure that is blocking the blood flow.

Congestion of the brain and nervous system

All blood from the brain also has to pass through the liver, be filtered of its toxins, and receive from the liver, a replenishment of all its nutritional needs. Toxins that don't get filtered out of the blood, stagnate in the brain. These toxins affect the brain in ways similar to the effects of alcohol.

Migraines and body aches and pains

Stagnated blood becomes toxic like the water of a blocked stream turning into a swamp. Over 90 percent of all aches and pains are caused by poisons or irritants that contact nerve endings. Pain indicates that the body is not handling or eliminating toxins and poisons as it must. They trigger a signal to the brain that warns the brain of their presence. Those that come in contact with brain cells cause pain felt as headaches. Wherever poisons stagnate and irritate nerve endings, they will create pain in those organs or areas.

Diabetes and Livers

The liver is the storehouse of body sugars. Any extra body needs, stress or stimulation, triggers the liver to dump more sugar back into the bloodstream. Excess sugar depletes insulin reserves and predisposes a person to diabetes.

About 80 percent of patients with fat saturated livers are pre-diabetic.

Liver Disease

Congestion Blockage of liver circulation	Decreased creation of proteins	Increased permeability of capillaries	Oxygen starvation of liver	Failure to control and balance hormones
Blocked flow of blood into liver	Low blood proteins	Leakage of proteins into tissues	Production of an anti-diuretic substance	
Increased (high) blood pressure	Decrease of blood osmotic pressure		Retention of sodium and water	Increased activity of a hormone called 'Aldosterone'

EDEMA

Escape of serum into tissues	Increased leg vein pressure		Increased blood pressure in veins	
				Decreased blood flow through the kidneys; less urine flow
General fluid swelling of tissues		Reduction of essential blood volume		Stimulation of adrenal glands & posterior pituitary

Caring for Your Liver

Without liver care and support, without a healthy liver there would be no health or total living, or being able to totally fulfill yourself.

The first approach to liver care is knowing, understanding and managing all possible hazards that damage the liver. There is no point in swallowing pills or liver restoring supplements, if little or no attention is paid to the causes of liver problems and to all its requirements. This means a careful avoidance of all toxins, body pollutants, chemicals and poisons. It means completely eliminating the stagnation of all of these.

The priority for liver therapy is to get the toxins, wastes, poisons, drugs and chemicals out of the body.

Important to the liver, as eating or any other therapy (their importance is in the order given below):

- Detoxify and eliminate liver hazards
- Positive attitudes, emotions and morale
- Joy of living through lifestyle
- Good regular exercise

- Clean, unpolluted air
- Alive, natural foods

Liver Detoxification Systems:

- Have as many bowel movements daily, as there are substantial meals. Whatever goes into the body must come out.
- Live with positive emotions, attitudes and lifestyle.
- Avoid all excesses.
- Maintain or activate a strong blood flow through the liver. This is the role of exercise, especially of deep breathing exercises.
- Avoid all lifestyle and habit excesses.
- In Chinese medicine, if one has too much anger it affects the liver. Also, suppressed anger may lead to depression.

If liver congestion has been a problem for a while, it is advisable to take supplements which act like liver flushes. Liver supplements made from beets that are grown in high zinc saturated soil are the most effective. Beets absorb great amounts of zinc as they grow. They create zinc enzymes. Zinc activates more enzyme systems in the liver and does more to increase liver efficiency than other minerals.

Natural, Detoxified Bile

Sluggish livers don't produce enough bile. Insufficient bile means inadequate elimination of liver poisons. Take as many bile tablets as required to completely restore the color of stools back to dark brown. (Cholacol is a detoxified bile supplement.)

Support your liver with nutrition

Our bodies and livers acquire the raw material they need to create their army of enzymes from what is in the foods we eat. By perfect nutrition, the liver generously provides every nutrient and elements required to rebuild all its cells, and make possible every function at optimal levels.

Our diets should include only live or undercooked (never microwaved or pressure cooked) chemically free, unadulterated foods, grown on naturally fertilized, completely mineralized soils. (No chemicals or pesticides).

Possibly, the best nourishment for livers is the livers from healthy animals. Only liver cells are sources of every molecule required for the perfect structure and functions of livers.

Unrefined, unprocessed supplements created from livers make excellent liver regenerating supplements.

Livers need and use large amounts of the Vitamin A and B complex group than any of the other vitamins. Livers suffer when deprived of these vitamin/enzyme teams.

Enzymes must be in and part of all foods. Supplements, to have healing powers, must be rich in enzymes. Liver enzymes must be in constant supply. Even a few hours of starvation lowers the vitality and functions of the liver.

Little about the role of enzymes in the liver, or in our bodies, is ever mentioned in medical books. They are practically never considered as medical therapies. They are not drugs. The use of enzymes as therapies would eliminate the need for almost all drugs. Enzymes cannot be manufactured by drug companies. Drug companies can make no profit from them. Their use would put drug companies out of business.

High Quality Protein Diets

The liver cannot subsist or function without a generous and constant supply of quality proteins, i.e., foods that provide all the amino acids in an excellent balance. A quality protein must be a part of every meal. One quarter of the daily food intake should be protein. Even a few hours of depriving the liver of proteins lowers its vitality and functions.

The proteins must always be in their natural nutrient forms. They must be foods that can be transformed into body and liver cells. Proteins must never be overcooked, chemically treated, hydrolyzed and liquefied or isolated into single amino acids.

Flesh meats, soybeans, millet are forms of high quantity (high concentration), but low quality, proteins. Excesses of these foods can overload and unbalance livers. When your liver is troubled, avoid them until it is well.

Proteins not only restore and sustain the liver, but satisfy and relieve hungers and cravings for excesses of foods, sweets, alcohol or cigarettes which could harm your liver.

Protein Excesses

It is also possible to overload our livers with proteins. Protein excesses place excess demands on liver enzyme reserves. They unbalancc the liver. When your liver is troubled, it is best for at least a couple of months, to avoid low quality/ high concentrate protein foods or supplements.

Proteins which contributes the most to a healthy liver:

- **Brewer's Yeast** is a liver tonic and protects the liver functions.
- **Seeds, grains** that are whole, soaked 48 hours and freshly ground.
- **Nuts** in shells, not roasted or salted. The best are almonds, hazelnuts and walnuts.
- **Deep ocean fish,** such as halibut, sole or salmon.
- **Eggs** from healthy, range fed and hen fertilized.
- **Methionine:** the liver needs and uses this amino acid to manufacturer choline and lecithin. Both of these are essential for the metabolism, transportation and mobilization of fats, oils, cholesterol and sterols, and for the production of hormones.
- **Internal organs**, such as liver, sweetbreads, heart, kidney from healthy, organically grown animals. To preserve their food value, prepare them by lightly broiling.

Animals of prey know about the value of livers. When a lion downs a prey, it first goes for and feasts on its liver.

If there is enough liver, it will not touch the muscle meats. It leaves these as leftovers for scavenger animals or birds. The values of the different nutrients show in the strength of the lion, compared to the weakness of the scavengers.

Quality Oil/Enzyme Complexes

Livers cannot function without oils, any more than a motor can. Our bodies and livers need two-to-three tablespoon servings daily. They are sources of essential oil-soluble vitamins. Oils trigger the flushing of the liver and the flow of bile with dissolved toxins.

Each oil contains more of certain nutrients than others. To get the most benefits, it is best to mix several kinds together. The most nutritious, essential and valuable oils are listed below:

- Avocados,
- Sesame seed, sunflower, safflower, flax, wheat germ oils
- Nuts, seeds, grains, cereals
- Internal organs
- Peanut or almond butter if made from freshly shelled, lightly roasted nuts

Certain oils provide therapeutic benefits in diseases caused by toxic oils or from a lack of hormones. They are...

Gamma Linolenic Acid

Many know Gamma Linolenic acid as primrose oil. It is also found in black currant. It plays an important role as the suit of "armor" protective coating for cell membranes and cell chromosomes. It reinforces the immune systems.

Choline

Choline is a fat dissolver, mobilizer and eliminator. Choline protects the liver against fatty degeneration. It transforms fat in the liver into lecithin and makes the fat soluble and transportable. Taking refined or process lecithin blocks this action.

Arachidonic Acid

An oil found in peanuts and sesame seeds is most essential to health. It benefits our body by contributing to the production of hormones. These are essential for maintaining healthy skin conditions and protecting against psoriasis, eczema, acne, dry scaly skin and dandruff, etc.

Livers require a variety of total foods that also include:

Juices. If you have a juicer, make your own juices

Vitamin A. Carrots, apples, beets (roots and leaves)

Vitamin B. Cucumbers, apples, dandelion leaves, fresh (organically grown, if possible)

Vegetables, fruits. The most beneficial to livers are...

- Salads (hot/cold) and a large variety of greens
- Baked potatoes and brown rice
- Carrots, beets, dandelion greens and radishes
- Parsley, celery, rhubarb, artichokes and endive
- Vegetable broths

Getting or preparing health restoring foods may be nearly impossible for people too ill to look after themselves. The best alternative is liver extract supplements in a pill form.

Liver Supplements – Food Concentrates

Thousands of companies sell vitamins and minerals in North America, but only a few produce products capable of restoring optimal health and function to livers. Such concentrates must not be heated. They must not be treated by chemicals. Their enzymes must have had no contact with air or oxygen. None of the liver restoring and healing enzymes must have been destroyed or lost, or extracted by the refining or processes of manufacturing. They must retain life force needed to replace those burned and used up light by livers in their fight against the pollutants of civilization.

Hepatrophin is a high food concentrate of complete liver extracts. It provides and replenishes all liver nutrients as required for perfect function and regeneration of liver structure and health.

Without zinc, selenium, sulphur and iron, the liver would be sluggish and is/or weak in its ability to repair damaged tissue, fight infection and detoxify the blood and bowel. The best source of zinc is in beet juice concentrates from beets grown on super-zinc saturated soils.

The best source of selenium is wheat germ and wheat germ oil. Selenium is an enzyme that forms the core of the Vitamin E complex, the major ingredient of wheat germ.

Exercise

Specifically deep breathing or diaphragmatic breathing exercises. The diaphragm works with a piston-like action. Its contractions put a downward pressure on the liver. The pressing down forces out the liver blood and the toxins it contains. When this diaphragmatic muscle relaxes, it releases pressure on the liver and allows it to expand. It draws it upward, creating a vacuum effect that pulls in increased amounts of blood with its contents of nutrients and toxins to be processed.

Breathe in as deeply as you can – without forcing. Hold for two to three seconds. Breathe in again – deeper. Hold your breath as long as you can comfortably. Slowly and gradually breathe out. This type of breathing is even more effective if done when trying to touch your toes, either while standing up or when sitting on the floor.

Sleep

Doctors of the past always demanded that patients get lots of bed rest. This was an essential part of good therapy. The liver needs rest and time to perform its functions.

Sleeping makes every therapy much more effective. Sleeping should be a part of every good liver health restoring program. Cutting back on the hours of sleep needed by an individual is to cut back on the hours the liver requires in order to break down and eliminate the waste and toxins accumulated in the previous days (or months) activities. The substances not handled will remain and accumulate in the liver. Getting lots of sleep is an important as other therapies for liver restoration.

Special therapies for liver support

Liver Flushes

To lubricate the bile ducts and to improve the functions of the whole liver, it is most beneficial to occasionally follow a detoxification regime and take two ounces of good quality oil mixed in a glass of grapefruit or orange juice.

Enemas

Enemas are valuable and often indispensable. They are especially so for those with serious or degenerative disease and who are in crisis states. They are indicated during periods when intense detoxification is indispensable.

Coffee enemas strongly stimulate and activate liver drainage. Caffeine accelerates the flushing out of liver toxins/wastes. Taken by rectum, the coffee goes directly to the liver. There it exerts a highly stimulating action.

Coffee enemas are prepared from only fresh ground coffee beans. The oils in stale coffee go rancid when they stand around a long time. Rancid oils are liver toxins.

Prepare the coffee by filter or percolator – in the same way as you prepare the beverage for drinking. Use 1 quart of ordinary strength coffee for each enema.

Pancreatic Enzymes

Almost before any other treatment is used, the completeness of digestion should be checked. The simple way to do this is by checking your bowel movements. If the digestion is perfect and complete, the stools will be well formed sausage shapes. They will be dark brown. No foods or food fragments or fibers will be invisible. There will be no holes in the stools. The stools will sink to the bottom of the toilet bowl. You will not pass any gas.

Fasting

I mention fasting here, although I've dedicated a full chapter to it. That's how important it is. Fasting is the most effective and "fast" way to decongest and flush out a liver and prevent further overloads and hazards. Leaving solid foods out of the diet allows the liver to use its reserves of enzyme to exclusively act on, break down and eliminate stagnant surpluses of body toxins and waste.

Avoid all solid foods for at least three to five days. Drink sweetened juices of grape, grapefruit or lemon, or drink herb teas with a little honey and lots of warm water (preferably distilled for a better absorption of toxins). After fasting, eat only fruits for a day or two. After add salads and vegetables, then back to a normal diet.

Liver detoxifying foods and herbs

- Apples, carrots, cucumbers and beets. If you have a juicer, drink the fresh squeezed extract from them.
- Watercress, nettles, nasturtium and alfalfa, garlic, onions and sea salt (as sources of minerals).
- Drink lots of liquids. They help to flush out toxic liver residues. Some liquids are capable of absorbing more toxins than others. They are:
    - Distilled water, unsweetened grape or grapefruit juices; lemon juice with warm water and unpasteurized honey.
- Juices made from the foods mentioned above – organically grown, if possible.
- Slippery Elm, Turkish Rhubarb, Pau d'Arco, Echinacea, Burdock, Yarrow, Goldenseal, Sheep Sorrel and Chaparral.
- Beverages include dandelion coffee, rosehips, sassafras and chamomile teas.
- Black radish herbs (in concentrates) is an excellent source of liver reinforcing and restoring enzymes.

- **Liver Restoring Herbs**

Historical records show that ancient Greeks used decoctions of milk thistle fruits as a liver remedy 2000 years ago. The Romans and doctors from India and Europe did so as well.

Milk Thistle

- Activates growth of new cells to replace damaged and dying cells and thereby help to renew the liver.
- Inhibits the viruses, alcohol, drugs, infections, carbon tetrachloride, allergens, mushroom poisonings and toxic chemicals that cause liver problems.
- Increases speed of synthesizing and utilizing proteins.
- Inhibits the oxygen molecules that break down oils. In diseased, inflamed livers, oxygen molecules, catalyzed by an enzyme called "lipoxygenase" create chemicals called "leukotrienes". These chemicals damage cells, block the production of liver enzymes, liver functions and the filtering of poisons from liver.
- Helps counteract or protect against many liver diseases disorders and damages.
- Slows down and builds resistance to cancer, especially when there are metastases to the liver from other areas.

The main active ingredients of milk thistle are:

- **Silymarin** is a bioactive compound. Ninety percent of it works in the liver cells. Silymarin prevents carbon tetrachloride, mushroom poisons, cigarette smoke, food additives, drugs and other foreign substances from damaging the liver. Silymarin reinforces the membrane structure of cells and block the passage of poisons in the liver cells. In similar ways, it protects the kidneys and prevents kidney damage.

- **Silybidin**, (the most active ingredient), silandrin and silyhermin protect cells from damage, including damage to the RNA, chromosomes and ribosome, which create the structures and functions of liver cells.

Reactions that can occur during therapy

Each effective therapy forces the healing processes of your liver to work even harder. The more effective the therapy, the greater the chances that you will experience, at some time, some discomforts or distresses that will upset you and cause you some anxiety. When livers react in such ways, they are working overly hard and over time. The reserves of healing and detoxifying enzymes have been exhausted. Your liver will complain or rebel by developing symptoms and distresses.

There is no organ that is more easily affected by external influences than the liver. The same as your liver is the most is the first organ to feel the effects of any toxicity, starvation or deficiency; it is the first to react to the benefits or side effects of a therapy.

Many changes or unusual feelings we experience are actually manifestations of our body's healing processes, of poisons or diseases leaving the body – much the same as a hangover after alcohol intoxication.

When unusual or unpleasant changes occur while taking remedies, we tend to assume that the remedy is not right for us and it is creating harmful side effects. When taking therapies that heal and are right for us, they create body changes. Whatever is experienced as a wrong is a "wrong" the body is attempting to get rid of. It is a "wrong" that is coming out; it is not a "wrong" of a remedy, or necessarily a wrong remedy.

We have been conditioned for many centuries to believe that every unusual and uncomfortable change in the ways our bodies are feeling or functioning is an evil. This is not always the case. There is an inborn wisdom in the body. Its ways and effects are sometimes unusual, even unpleasant, but our bodies make no mistakes.

These distresses are called “Healing Reactions”

Whenever you carefully follow a regime that has been tailored to your healing needs, and you experience what seems to be a setback or an unpleasant reaction, your body may be telling you that it is working beyond its abilities. It needs a rest; it needs time to catch up with its overloads. Rather than getting upset, or anxious, take a short holiday from your treatment. Give your liver a break. Stop supplements that make your liver work harder. Increase those that help to ease the liver congestion and overload. Consult your holistic physician to know how to do this.

When one experiences adverse reaction is the time to consider fasting, as described above.

You should experience some relief within a few days. Taking liver supplements will accelerate to this.

Allow your body to experience feeling good again, for at least two days. Then resume your prescribed regime.

How long do our livers need special care?

A rough estimate is about one year of therapy for every 10 years of illness, problems and liver abusing. Liver precautions must be carefully and constantly followed until health is restored.

Counsels

The most important service one can provide for health protection and prevention of disease is to provide an abundance of tender loving care for our livers. Never treat your liver lightly. It cannot be replaced. Learn to love your liver. Give your liver a break.

To keep your liver healthy is to keep your whole body in a state of optimum health. If your liver goes, so does health, immunity, vigor, healing, emotional and physical wellbeing and peace of mind.

Learn to live close to Mother Nature and by her laws. Nothing that man can do will ever improve on what the Creator abundantly provides for us in nature.

Eliminate what is negative, artificial and/or denatured. Restore or maintain positive attitudes, emotions and lifestyles. Health does not depend only on your physician. Health also and always depends on you.

Liver care is healthcare,

Life care,

Optimal living.

Get lots of rest, fresh air and exercise,

Eat only fresh, alive foods,

Don't hurry – don't worry

Live your life to the fullest

Live positively, peacefully debt – joyfully

The Gallbladder and Liver Flush

The following protocol can be used with or without the use of enemas to clean, deodorize and heal the digestive tract.

This program has been taken in part from the book: *Health Questions and Answers* by Alan Nittler, M.D.

1. Combine the juice of either one orange, grapefruit, lemon. You can also mix two or all of them together with extra virgin cold pressed olive oil. Make 1 ½ ounces or 1/8th of a cup.
2. Blend well together by placing the liquid in a closed jar or container and shake well for about 30 seconds.
3. Take the mixture for five consecutive evenings.
4. Rest for two evenings. Repeat for another five evenings. You can drink it before bedtime. If preferred, it works equally well if taken in the morning in place of your breakfast.
5. Consume no food until noon.

6. A hot herbal beverage, such as chamomile tea helps tremendously to intensify the cleansing action of the formula.

See below the following recommended herbs to cleanse and to strengthen the detoxifying functions of the gallbladder, liver and digestive organs.

Herb Name	Number of Tables to be taken		
	Breakfast	Lunch	Daily Total
Lidan G.B. Cleanse	4-5	4-5	8-10
Shu Kan Liver Cleanse	6-8	6-8	12-16
Garlic (non-odor type) to flush toxins	2-3	2-3	4-6
Acidophilus Yeast (to normalize bowel flora)	2-3	2-3	4-6

After the first few days on the above detoxification program, you should become aware of...

- A marked enhancement of your energy and restoration of your vitality and reserves.
- This program can provoke a mild, temporary diarrhea. This is beneficial and should not be taken as a problem or a reason for your concern.

For continued improvement of body detoxification and health:

- Drink eight to 10 glasses or more of distilled water per day
- Chamomile tea offers special benefits to gallbladders and their function.

- Four to five glasses of apple and/or grape juice daily, diluted 50 percent with distilled water.
- A diet of 75 percent (undercooked) vegetables and fruits.
- Restricting intake of tea, coffee, soft drinks and alcohol.
- Eliminating cigarettes, drugs, fats, refined sugars and foods, and junk food.
- Dead, refined and chemically treated foods.

Your follow-up to the above detoxification program is determined by the understanding of the causes of your health problems brought to light by your case history and your doctor's interpretation.

Fasting for Lasting Heath

If you have never tried fasting, you haven't experienced real health and revitalization. You haven't enjoyed the pleasures of renewed vitality, exhilaration and exuberance.

The first time that you go on a fast you will regret that you hadn't done it sooner. – Dr. Leo Roy, MD

Fasting is an exhilarating experience in health restoration.

Fasting...

- Hastens pain relief.
- Promotes more rapid elimination of toxins.
- Prepares the body so that it can undertake the task of total rebuilding and restoration.

We are conditioned since childhood to believe that to miss even one meal is not good for our health. It is harmful. The mere thought of depriving oneself of food is not to be considered by anyone in their right mind. It is so important to keep up our energy. Surely the more foods we eat the more healthy we will be. Those home-cooked meals taste so good: "Come on, have another helping. You need to eat more. You are a growing boy/girl".

Such ways of looking at fasting disregards the reality that....

- Body organs and biochemistry need rest just as much as they need nutrition.
- Our bodies can only use the nutrition needed to perform their daily functions. More than that overloads them and clog up tissues and use of valuable energy reserves.
- Bodies have to do the work to breakdown and get rid of excesses.
- Food excesses do not increase physical, mental or emotional strengths. They hamper and make sluggish our abilities to live our optimal best.
- Balance is essential to health as is abundance.

Experiments on test animals have shown that feeding them only the exact amounts they need to keep active without losing weight, can actually double their lifespan. Food excesses cause health problems.

Dietary moderation is a major factor for optimal health.

When eating, there comes a moment when we feel satisfied. We don't really need any more food. Our brain even send signals telling us this. Too often we listen to our appetites and desires for gratification rather than to our brain.

When we disregard the wisdom of our mind and continue to indulge in excesses, our brain still tries to help us by turning off our appetites. If brains could talk, we would hear the message:

"Food excesses harm. Stop eating. Give me a chance to clear out useless, detrimental excesses and get caught up with the work of living that I need to do. Your excesses are clogging up your organs. Bodies cannot maintain their performance of excellence when overloaded."

Food excesses threaten health and hinder healing

Most of us consume great excesses of food and drink. We pay no attention to the accumulations of waste and "garbage" in our bodies. So what? We will use it up by exercising.

If you have never lived free of this garbage and pollution, you have never experienced the exhilaration, the vitality, the wellbeing, the enthusiasm of real living. You have never enjoyed the pleasures of really being and completely your real self. You have never experienced the flourishing of your potentials. To have lived without detoxifying and fasting and lived in moderation, is to have deprived yourself of a most valuable means of maintaining health and of healing. You may never realize all your worth until you have revitalized your body by careful and wise fasting.

Fasting is not a form of self-punishment. It is a blessing.

Fasting...

- Gives our body a rest from excesses and abuses we have imposed upon it.
- Allows our body to break down, decompose and burn up accumulated body wastes, inadequately digested foods, deposits of fat, sick, dying and abnormal cells, toxic chemicals, body pollutants, abscesses, tumors and even allergens.

- Gives our bodies a chance to eliminate and flush out toxic wastes, debris and pollutants. It is our bodies most effective and quickest way of doing this. It is a spring cleaning job.
- Eliminates barriers and hindrances to regenerate and heal.
- Spares body energies. Twenty five percent of all the energies we use each day are required for digestion. Resting our digestive organs allows the body to reroute those energies for healing.
- Is the ideal way for 'kicking' habits and addictions for drugs, alcohol and smoking.
- Is the perfect protection against disease.
- Creates conditions that allow our bodies to restore themselves to their original state of excellence.
- Rests our organs of digestion so that they can be revitalized and be restored to their optimum health and function.
- Restores, regenerates and revitalizes high-level wellbeing to our bodies, minds, emotions and spirits, and to all of our living.
- Is an indispensable part of living and healing.
- Is natural to all living beings. Even dumb (or not so dumb) animals are smart enough to quit eating when they are ill or traumatized. Fasting repels only those who live for self-indulgence – who can't tolerate thoughts of depriving themselves of their gratifications of eating.
- Fasting prepares our bodies for the feasting of real living.

Millions of cells die every minute of our lives. Our normal activities of wear and tear destroy up to three billion cells every day. They die, they decompose and they become toxic microscopic cadavers. For many of us, our foods do not completely digest. Food that is not completely digested, rots, putrefies or ferments. It turns into toxic substances. The debris of poorly digested, poor quality, and dead foods accumulate and stagnate as pollutants. They are like ashes from a burned out fire or exhaust fumes from a motor.

Unless completely broken down and eliminated, they become putrefying garbage.

Even when free of diseases and still considered to be healthy, our bodies harbor pounds of toxins. Everything that has not been transformed into what the body's biochemistry and organs can use is virtually poison. We live in a state of toxicity. We too often take for granted that the fatigues, distresses and discomfort caused by all the spotty toxicity is inevitable or even a normal part of our nature, and all of our living. Not so.

This is living without knowing what it is like to be healthy. In the midst of all the abnormal conditions of our civilization, we do not, and cannot, know the exhilaration of peak health. Until we free ourselves from these toxic relations, until we start fasting, we may never achieve this realization.

To better understand this we need to know the nature of toxins that affect us and how they affect us.

Bowel wastes

Fecal matter is made up of all the end products of digestion, the residues of foods and/or other substances which we have ingested, but have not been of any use, plus the billions of cadavers of cells that die each day.

Undigested foods putrefy or ferment in the bowel. It forms gas. This gas can be toxic as small doses of arsenic. Gas, plus the stagnating toxic bowel wastes and chemicals, react with the tissues that make the walls in the muscles of our intestines. The drugged muscles of the intestinal walls lose their ability to contract and discharge their loads, at least not as often, or as well as is needed to keep the bowels clean and free of poisons.

Some of the retained poisons succeed in filtering through the intestinal wall. They become a major factor in body toxicity.

Fatigue Poisons

Stresses, excesses and abuses wear out cells and accelerate and increase the number that die every minute. The dead and abnormal biochemical that come from these dying cells accumulate in the fluids and in the spaces between all cells in our tissues. They overload and overtax the liver and other toxin processing organs.

Emotional Toxins

Traumas, grief, anger, hatred, fears, worries, all strong negative feelings, thoughts and attitudes, affect and denature the biochemical throughout our body. They too create toxins.

Pollutants

In our "civilized" living, we absorb almost everything we breathe, drink and eat, chemicals, preservatives, pesticides, colorings, artificial flavors, thickeners, sweeteners, additives and the industrial and environmental pollutants. Thousands of them are so toxic that they contribute to cancer.

Body residues of diseases of earlier years

The elements which caused such illnesses, as well as all the drugs used to control them, remain in our body's storage spaces. They are never completely eliminated.

Ways our bodies have of detoxifying and eliminating toxins, debris and poisons

Understanding the ways of detoxifying is a big part of understanding the importance of fasting and how fasting works.

Ninety five percent of all poisons come into the body, via our mouths. They are in commercial foods, non-foods, junk foods, fast foods, overcooked foods, microwave foods, processed and refined foods, synthetic and artificial foods, nonfood form beverages, soft drinks, alcohol, pills, drugs, cigarettes and on, and on.

Almost invariably, at least a small portion of poisons filter through the intestines and into our blood. They are carried to our liver. The liver is the body's main poison-handling-and-disposal-processing organ. It chemically neutralizes, annihilates and disintegrates almost everything that our bodies don't like and can't use. These are then put into a solution in bile. The bile carries everything to the intestines to be flushed out and eliminated.

Water-soluble toxins and poisons go to the kidneys where they are flushed out in the urine. Some poisons get burned up like wood on a fire. The residues from this "burning" are gases like carbon dioxide and they go to the lungs, which exhale them out. Some toxins - those which are minerals - pass out of the body by our perspiration – through the skin.

Non-eliminated poisons stagnate in the blood. The blood carries them out through our tissues and cells – anywhere and everywhere. They find ways to infiltrate the tissues and hide, and store there. The main storage tissues are fat cells – body fat.

Some toxic minerals stay in the blood. They travel to our brain where they generate toxicity and the symptoms that signal their presence. Some contact nerve endings in our tissues and these nerves are warning signals to your brain. More symptoms are created, all of which indicate the presence and excesses of threatening and harmful chemicals.

The role of nerves is to notify you in some way that the wellness of those tissues or areas of the body is being threatened by an abnormal substance, chemical or poison. They have no words by which to speak to the brain or us. They speak with red warning flags, such as pain, headaches, hangovers and the symptoms listed below.

- The body feels like it's going through a hangover
- Fevers, infections
- Colds, flues
- Abscesses, oils, pimples, skin diseases
- Body odor, bad breath, foul odor of feces/urine
- Darkened urine
- Coated tongue
- Fatigue, exhaustion, sluggishness
- Lack of drive and ambition
- Loss of libido and sex drive
- Weakness, debility
- Decreased thinking abilities, concentration
- Failing memory

- Depression, demoralization
- Easily upset nerves and emotions, irritability
- Sleeping difficulties, agitated dreams, nightmares
- Headaches, heavy head
- Aches, pains, cramps
- Nausea, stomach sickness
- Vomiting, diarrhea
- Allergy conditions
- Overweight, difficulties in losing the weight
- Decrease of body functions
- Decrease of our natural healing abilities
- Being afflicted by a serious, degenerative disease or chronic condition

All strong reactions to drugs, chemicals and poisons are hangovers. Bodies go through hangovers from all poisons and pollutants – not just when it is "drying out" from alcohol or drugs from the "morning after the night before." Hangovers are a normal healing process.

Bodies react to and fight poisons. They flush them out of our tissues. They bring them into our blood streams. The blood goes promptly to the brain. The brain becomes toxic – poisoned. We feel terrible.

Fasting is detoxification

Detoxification is ridding our bodies of any and every abnormal substance or excess. Fasting is sometimes the only way our bodies can detoxify quickly and effectively enough to prevent serious consequences and illness to our bodies integrity and perfection.

Fasting is the most effective, fastest method of detoxification

We all need to go on fasts. Those with serious illnesses need them badly. The contaminants and pollutants of our air, water and food, have over our lifetimes greatly overloaded our organs of detoxification and elimination.

Depending on the severity of an illness, a five-to-seven day (or longer) fast, at least two-to-four times a year is recommended. Longer is even better, if you can remain comfortable while on it.

We cannot eat and detoxify at the same time. Just like we cannot fill a jar with water and empty it at the same time. Eating is like having the jar of our bodies in the upright position. Fasting is like turning the jar upside down.

Several conditions are required by the body in order to detoxify and eliminate.

The requirements are...

- Freeing the detoxification and elimination organs from their need to work on other substances so that they can process toxic wastes and get them out of our bodies. This is done by refraining from putting foods or solids in our systems to be worked on by those organs.
- Resting our bodies and maintaining these organs in peak condition by sustaining and replenishing their energies and enzymes.
- Providing the body with plentiful fluids to enable it to carry all the waste and poisons out of the body.
- Allowing the body all the days it needs to complete its task of breaking down and eliminating all the poisons and restoring itself to a state of optimal wellbeing.

Fasting is ingesting only liquids and avoiding solid foods

There are different ways of fasting. For instance, one can fast...

- By following rigid principles.
- In a negative, sacrificial way of "poor me" by forcing.

Or by...

- Wanting to be good to your body.
- Listening to your body's every need.
- Catering to your body's needs in beneficial ways.

- Enjoying a preferable experience.

Before Fasting

Make sure you understand what you must do, how to do it, what to expect. In case difficulties or problems arise, it is best to know about them beforehand. Ignorance could leave you concerned and upset. This could influence you to pursue your fast in ways that are not right for you. Carefully read and understand the contents of this book.

To the best of your abilities...

- Unload worries, anxieties, concerns, fears and mental, physical, and emotional distresses – everything that might upset you.
- Take supplements and food concentrates you need to satisfy all deficiency needs and compensate for any, and every weakness.
- Eliminate for several days before fasting, all stimulants: caffeine, cigarettes, alcohol, processed, instant and overcooked foods, desserts, soft drinks, processed non-foods forms, vitamins, minerals, amino acids or supplements in liquid, hydrolyzed, refined forms and single amino acids.
- Avoid lifestyle excesses, habits. Live a reasonable lifestyle. Be aware of, and don't treat lightly, any serious illness that might be present in your system.
- Abstain from drugs, pills and chemicals. Taking any of these for health problems, should be discussed with the doctor you use to guide your fast.
- Follow a preparation period of at least two-to-three weeks. For first-time fasters, this is very important.
- Eat only undercooked or raw foods for one or two days prior to fasting: salads, soups, fresh fruits, vegetables, etc.
- Avoid meats, overcooked foods, highly spicy foods, sugars, fats, fried foods, starches and desserts.

- Drink only spring or demineralized water. Take enough to satisfy your thirst. A little extra adds to the body's ability to flush out more toxins and wastes.
- Ease into fasting **gradually**. Never, ever force any aspect of fasting.

Many books on fasting claim that there is only one way to fast, one way that works, and that is usually their way. There are various and many ways of fasting. They all work. There are no rigid, law-bound, stereotype systems or methods that apply to every person under all circumstances. As long as you detoxify, your fast is a good one.

Starting your Fasts

During the week prior to fasting, prepare yourself by taking three days of juices and one day of solids: vegetables, salads, fruits, nuts, grains. Or, two days of juices and one day of solids: vegetables, salads, fruits, nuts and grains.

Preliminary 24-hour: A Trial Fast

This involves merely avoiding food from supper one day until supper the next day, taking no solid foods for breakfast or lunch – missing only two meals. For those fasting for the first time, this is usually the best way to begin. You tend to feel poorly, or get a headache sometimes during the end of 24 hours. As soon as you feel it is too difficult to go on, being without food is an ordeal (this is not for me) or a headache becomes severe, stop. There is no need to force. Forcing never does anybody any good. There is always next week to try again.

It can take one, two or three tries before a body feels able to tolerate the lack of food. After the trial fast that is not too difficult, is the time to continue on with the full fast.

During the weeks between trial fasts, it is best to restrict diet to natural foods, undercooked foods, salads, fruits, nuts and whole grain cereals and make sure to have plentiful bowel eliminations. Take herbal laxatives if necessary.

Alternate ways of fasting.

Short Fasts

There is the once a week day of rest from food – a "Sabbath" is a most excellent practice.

Fasts of three-to-seven days can be done any time with confidence. They can be repeated, but preferably not more frequently than every six-to-eight weeks.

Long Fasts: Fasts of 15-to-40 days

If planning a long fast, obtain counsel and/or guidance. Have access to, and communicate with, a holistic physician in case any reactions occur or special needs arise.

Before undertaking serious long fasts, and to eliminate all possibilities of reactions, problems or complications, you should have your health evaluated to assure you there is no...

- Insufficiency of energy reserves.
- Inefficiencies of organs of eliminations – bowels.
- Inadequacies of liver, kidneys, pancreas or of other organs that break down and eliminate poisons.
- Endocrine glands imbalances and/or inadequacies.
- Problems with the functions of any organs.
- Deficiencies of proteins, oils, minerals, enzymes and/or vitamins.
- Imbalances of acid or alkaline reserves, especially excesses of acidity.

Fasting Advice: precautions during fasting

- Maintain normal mental and daily life activities. Fasting does not require making serious or radical lifestyle changes.
- Don't blindly follow this information or any system or book on fasting. Use this book or other books only as guidelines. Follow your body and what it tries to tell you. Changes,

discomforts and reactions indicate your body needs that must be understood and cared for. Let your doctor help you interpret them.

- It is important that you fast with confidence and reassurance.
- Don't predetermine the length of time you will stay on a fast. Only your body knows how long you can fast with benefit. Only your body knows what quantities of poisons and wastes it can handle before becoming tired or depleted. Your body's needs will indicate to you how long to continue and when to break off the fast. Learn to listen to your body.
- Increase bowel elimination. Maintain daily elimination during the period of fasting. Never go longer than one day without one good bowel movement. Even when no food is eaten, tissues continue to break down and need to be eliminated. Bowel stagnation increases toxicity, blocks healing and defeats the purpose of fasting.
- If necessary, take an herbal laxative, especially if you have been constipated for a number of years; i.e., having less quantities of bowel elimination than quantity of daily food intake.

Use any of the following liquids:

Spring, demineralized (reverse osmosis or distilled) water. Use whenever thirsty – as much as desired. Distilled water dissolves and flushes out more of the body toxins than do the mineral-saturated or spring waters.

Lemon juice, freshly squeezed, one-to-two teaspoons in a glass of water. Add unpasteurized honey, up to one teaspoon according to taste or grape, papaya, carrot, apple, orange, grapefruit. These are better taken diluted, 50/50 with demineralized water.

Juices are best when freshly extracted through a juicer. Drink juices at room temperatures, not ice cold or hot. Use not more than four-to-five glasses daily.

Juices provide...

- **Minerals** that alkalize, neutralize body acids.
- **Nutrients** that bypass the need for digestion and go rapidly into the bloodstream and the body.
- **Elements and enzymes** required for better detoxification and elimination.

  N.B: Frozen juices and from concentrates, for example, *V8 and Garden Cocktail* contain some undesirable substances. Use only when nothing else is available.

- **Herbal Teas**
  - Peppermint and Chamomile promote digestive enzymes secretion. These enzymes contribute to the breakdown of food and body wastes.
  - Fenugreek dissolves and flushes out mucus excesses and their content of body wastes. Optional: add a little natural honey and/or a little lemon juice. Herb teas are best when made with demineralized water.

Many books on fasting restrict everything except water. This may have been acceptable in years past. People lived closer to nature than we do now. They lived on quality food, air and water. They had stronger heredities, vital energy reserves and basic good health.

In our generation, people often are too exhausted and too depleted to fast without the support of extra nutrients and life energies. Our civilized and polluted living leaves us without the same vital health reserves. All who have had health problems or who have specials health needs, should take some such supplements during fasting.

Deficiencies in our organs of detoxification and elimination reduce our body's abilities to rid itself of its toxins. To provide no support during fasting, other than water, deprives the body of elements and energies essential for optimal functioning of these organs.

Small amounts of natural, unrefined sugar-containing foods (fruits, honey) are important in fasting. Taking them can turn a fast that would be detrimental and depleting, into one that is beneficial, restoring and revitalizing.

They do not "break the fasts" by interfering with or decreasing the detoxifying processes. To the contrary, they increase the body's abilities to detoxify. The liver needs sugars in order to perform its enormous task of getting rid of toxins. Your brain needs and uses as much sugar as the rest of the whole body. Low sugar levels can rob you of support and benefits you need during fasting. You go low. Feeling low could prompt you to want to quit.

Sugars in juices and honey provide fuel for the organs of elimination. Sugars are part of the biochemical mechanism for burning up fats and toxins; inadequately broken down fats turn into acids and "ketones". Acids and ketones are toxic and irritating to the nervous system. They are causes of possible dangers or complications of fasting. They cause nervous problems sometimes experienced during fasting. By maintaining efficient detoxification and keeping up the body's energies one can stay on the fasts for longer time. This allows for increased elimination of toxins.

The alkaline minerals in fruit and vegetable juices, or in special food concentrates, maintain nutritional and energy reserves. They offset the formation and buildup of assets and ketones. Other food concentrates or supplements also have the abilities to do this.

Supplements during Fasting

The use of food concentrates provide comfortable and effective revitalizing, gratifying, health-producing fasting. This does not include using common vitamins and minerals.

Some of the best food concentrates are:

- Bee pollen, ginseng, royal jelly and product formulations, which contain these.
- The vacuum dehydrated juices of sprouted wheat. These are man's perfect foods. These provide all body nutrients,

> as well as the life forces to maintain high levels of body energies. They do not interfere with the body's detoxifying mechanisms, but markedly enhance them.

Taking natural products when fasting, keeps up the body's energies and satisfies all needs for nutrients so wonderfully that after a few days on the fast you feel completely comfortable. You hardly know you are fasting. You feel great; you feel you could go on and on.

There are other supplements which do a marvelous job of flushing toxins from the liver, absorbing the poisons while they are in the intestines, so that they do not stagnate and increase the overall toxic elimination.

The first and most obvious of course are:

Herbal Laxative

There are many herbal laxatives available from herbal and health product distributors. Which ones are best for you? Only your body knows. They are the ones which produce the most bowel movements without causing cramps or discomfort. You will have to try one or another until you recognize the kind that helps you the most.

Avoid prune juice as a laxative during fasts. It is too acid forming. Fasting is already conducive to forming too many acids.

Toxin and Pollutant Absorbers and Adsorbers

There are products which bind to themselves, the molecules of chemicals, drugs and toxic substances and carry them out of the body by means of the bowel movements. They act almost like ravenous sponges. They have no chemical action or effect on the body. They remove harmful bacteria from the intestines.

They add bulk to the bowel movements. Two of the most effective of these are the Yucca herbs and Bentonite.

Yucca

A most effective, detoxifying herb. It coats and protects the intestinal skin lining, preventing the absorption of toxins into the body. It carries out of the intestines great amounts of toxic substances.

Bentonite

It absorbs intestinal bacteria and viruses. It can bind and carry out of the body up to 200 times its weight of harmful substances. Bentonite binds to itself the debris of billions of cells which die every day. It quickly relieves the symptoms of abdominal cramps, headaches, nausea and weakness. There are no side effects. It is best taken with psyllium seed. Flax seed and other fiber products also help.

Digestive Enzymes

It is the role of digestive enzymes to handle the majority of body wastes and pollutants. When these are in insufficient amounts, we become toxic.

The stomach and pancreas of many people do not secrete amounts of enzymes sufficient enough to completely disintegrate, neutralize and eliminate total toxic waste. This problem is more noticeable as age increases. Fasting under these conditions is not beneficial as it should be. It is important that such people take digestive enzyme supplements, either those of the stomach or those of the pancreas, or both.

How can one know which to take and how many to take? There are no stereotyped answers that apply to all individuals. Everybody is different; however, answers are readily provided by looking at your stools. If they're perfectly well formed, firm, dark brown, smooth surface, and sausage -shaped, formations without holes, or visible fibers or fragments of foods, they sink, and you experience no intestinal gas, you do not have a digestion or detoxification problem. Any deviation from these criteria indicates that you need extra enzymes.

In the next chapter, the importance of enzymes will be discussed in more detail. A full spectrum enzyme supplement should contain enzymes that breakdown proteins, fats, carbohydrates, fiber and milk sugars.

Here is a sample of a full spectrum digestive system enzyme capsule:

- Pancreatic protease with acid stable protease, breaks down protein.
- Lipase breaks down fats
- Alpha amylase, breaks down carbohydrates
- Amyloglucosidase breaks down carbohydrates
- Cellulase breaks down fibre
- Hemicellulase breaks down fibre
- Lactase breaks down milk sugar (is a type of carbohydrate)

Excellent food sources for enzymes: The aspergillus plant, avocados, bananas, papaya (papain, pineapple (bromelain), mangoes, sprouts. Papain and bromelain are protein digesting enzymes (proteases).

Fasting and Livers

Our livers perform most of the functions of purifying our blood, detoxifying our system and eliminating all body's poisons.

We all have a liver problem. It is not possible to live in our cities and polluted environment for two-to-four generations, to overcome the abnormal conditions of civilization. Our chemically processed and polluted foods, water and air; the excesses of radiation, our stresses, distresses and lifestyle excesses and still have a perfectly functioning liver, especially if there have been periods of ill health and exhaustion. Liver problems do not necessarily mean liver disease. It usually means the liver enzyme systems are deficient.

During fasting, excesses of toxic substances can very much overload the liver. Your liver is as tired as you feel. A lack of energy reserve is the main reason for liver fatigue. It loses its ability to perform its role as the body's main detoxifier.

Some of the best products to restore and retain optimum liver functions are:

- Concentrated liver regenerating extracts. (Hepatropfin – Standard Process)
- Beet juice (V. E. Irons) or Betafood Standard Process and/or Black Radish, (both standard process). These are enzymes which decongest and flush out all liver wastes and toxins.
- Other herbal liver flushes and supports are: Milk Thistle, Dandelion roots, Burdock.
- Bile tablets. (Cholacol or Cholacol 11 – S.P.). Bile is the liquid which flushes out and carries away the liver wastes and toxins into the intestines. It is also a laxative.
- Pale colored stools and craving for sweets are the indications that tell us we need bile. If bothered during a fast, take two-to-three tablets a day. Take enough to restore a dark brown color to your stools.
- Acidophilus (Mycelium/Lactic Acid yeasts) or yogurt wafers. Each time wind passes, a wafer should be taken. Take as many wafers as required to be completely free of gas.
- Intestinal gas is common. When it stagnates in the bowel, it is toxic and damaging to the body. This decreases bowel elimination. Gas reabsorbs into the body. Body toxicity increases. Neutralizing toxic gas is important during fasting.

Fasting Discomfort and Upsets

Distresses or discomforts experienced when not eating do not usually come on because of lack of food. They are from the toxins that have built up in your body over years which are beyond your body's ability to handle.

It is almost normal to expect some abnormal feelings during fasts, especially for toxin saturated people fasting for the first time.

Serious reactions, discomforts, pain or complications are NOT common.

Shortly after food intake is cut off, the body switches gear. It first needs after sustaining itself with nutrients is to get rid of any and all toxic substances, which threaten its wellbeing. It promptly starts to do this.

Its mechanisms bring to the surface all body wastes, stored toxins and abnormal elements. These re-enter the bloodstream. They contact the nerves, which are everywhere. Our bodies react to toxins coming from our storage areas the same as it does to poisons we take into our system by mouth or from outside the body.

All reactions indicate that toxic residues are excessive.
Fasting reactions generally occur, if one has prepared his/her body properly and adequately. Otherwise there are...

- Weaknesses or fatigue.
- Hungers: severe at first then declining up to two-to-four days. Then there is feelings of very little hunger until the body's tolerance limit has been reached. It is promptly relieved by consuming juice.
- "Hangover" toxic feelings: discomforts as described earlier.
- Dizziness, faintness, fatigue, weakness. These are to be expected when blood sugars get low. They are promptly relieved by a teaspoon of honey or by a glass of fruit juice.
- Coated tongue: white, yellow or brown. Tongues indicate the detoxifying process is in action.
- Dry mouth and foul breath. These are odors that come from poorly digested, putrid substances that were not eliminated from an uptight spastic intestines.
- Constipation. It is not unusual to not have a daily bowel movement during fasting, especially after the second or third day. It is best to relieve this by laxatives or enemas.

Experiencing reactions or discomfort does not mean that fasting is not for you or that you should cease your fast. Almost always the unpleasant feelings are caused by your body's pouring back into your bloodstream poisons from their storage areas. Your body is detoxifying. There is so much poison that has to be dumped from your body that you're feeling poisoned.

The more severe the reactions when going without food, the greater are your needs for a thorough cleansing; the greater is your need for a really good fast.

Handling and Controlling Reactions

As a band-aid, these unpleasant distresses can be halted promptly by going back on to food. This is the same as taking alcohol when having a hangover. Taking food into your body stops the reactions of fasting. The foods and alcohol merely stop the body from dumping its poisons back into your blood. As stated earlier, the body can't do both at the same time. The relief you experience still does not mean that your discomforts are caused by a lack of food, nor does it mean that taking food is compensating for a body need. The discomforts of fasting have ceased by going off the fast, but so has the whole process of detoxification and elimination. The toxins have merely been pushed back into their original storage spaces and you don't feel their effects anymore. Your body remains toxic.

Some reactions and upsets are non-toxic

Weakness and fatigue occur when the body and blood sugar become depleted. Taking a glass of fruit juice or lemon juice and honey provides prompt relief. A sense of a pickup usually follows. The relief confirms that the low blood fuel levels were the only factor responsible for these discomforts.

Weight Loss

When pounds are lost, some people get scared. It is important to realize that what appears to be a weight lost is almost totally only the loss of toxic debris, pollutants and water. The greater the loss of these, the better off you are.

A loss of weight is not to be feared from short fasts. Those up to one or two weeks. Possibly only a pound or more of actual body flash is really lost. This small amount of flash is replaced by your eating in the weeks that follow. A healthy body always tends to seek its normal and perfect weight. If you're underweight, the same applies.

Healing Crises and Toxic Reactions

If any occur, don't panic or become unduly concerned. Fasting and detoxification processes are most or all of these distresses.

Most reactions are easily handled by:

- Taking laxatives or enemas. Use whenever the bowel elimination is inadequate. Take as many as are required to bring about complete relief, comfort and the return of your sense of wellbeing.
- Increasing the supplements already listed.

If the reaction you experience is not serious, it is usually advisable to just ignore it for a day or so, while trying the above suggestions.

If any distress persists or intensifies, simply discontinue the fast. Go back on food. Start again at a later date. Assuming you are not in a serious disease state, there is no real need to force the fast beyond its endurance. There is no urgency to rapidly restore your health. Let your body heal itself at its own pace, in its own way, in its own ability.

Determining how long to fast

There is no simple answers or stereotyped guidelines for knowing when to break the fast. The fasting time varies with each individual. Only your body knows the extent of its ability to handle its toxins and fast. It alone knows how long it can go without food.

If body changes, messages, signs and symptoms leave you concerned, worried or confused, get your holistic physician to interpret them for you. There is no harm in stopping your fast when you are feeling great. However, by quitting too soon, you may miss a lot of the healing benefits and sheer exhilaration may be short lasting.

Indications that a fast has accomplished its purpose

You have spent days free of hunger, fatigue and toxic feelings. You have experienced alertness, a sharp mind, a clear head and a lightness. You feel no more need for food. Your tongue and breath have cleared. (The tongue does not always clear completely; the edges turn pink.) The breath sweetens. Your good feelings have reached a plateau. You have enjoyed them for a number of days. Everything seems steady and stable.

It is best not to stop fasting when you are feeling good and on a high. Feeling good is your body telling you to keep right on doing with what you've been doing. You are still doing fine. It is the right thing to do. Please, don't stop.

Then, one morning you wake up not feeling so great. You feel tired again; a little draggy. You may even start to feel poorly or "punk". Your thoughts start dreaming of food. In your sleep you may have dreamt about a steak, or your favorite food. You could eat a bear, even one on the run.

These changes can occur only after a few days or after a good number of days. Your body wisdom knows when you have detoxified as much as you can and you need a rest from this. You've had enough. It is time to stop fasting. It is time to eat again. Ring the dinner bell. Bring on the chow!

But, you can stop too soon

To stop fasting prematurely is to block an elimination of poisons and wastes that your body still feels a need to get rid of. If you start eating again before these poisons have been eliminated, you will again experience toxicity, discomfort and/or fatigue feelings.

If after stopping your fast, in the days that follow, you experience letdowns, lows, or discomforts; your body is telling you that there are still free floating poisons in your blood. You should have gotten rid of them and didn't. It would be best for you to restart your fast and continue until you experience the indications to stop.

Proper ways to break the fast

- First phase: eat mainly fruits. Preferably, cherries, oranges, grapefruits, apples, pineapples or fruits that you crave are particularly desire. Each one every four to five hours. Stewed prunes help for good bowel movements. For every four to five days of fasting do one day on fruits.
- Second phase: add soups: vegetables, salads, spinach and greens. Lightly cooked leafy vegetables. Temporarily avoid the starchy, root vegetables. One or two days are all your body needs to adapting.
- Third phase: add nuts, grains, cereals, starches and root vegetables and/or any particular quality food for which you experience a special craving, for another one to three days.
- Fourth phase: back to a normal diet, but do not return to those overcooked, dead, devitalized, junk foods, fast foods, canned foods, TV dinners, fried foods, etc. – those which contributed to your toxicity in the first place. To go back to your old ways, will rob you of all the benefits you received from your fasting.

"It is a mistake to believe that fasting cures diseases. Wrong living and excesses create disease. Fasting does not, cannot cure errors of living, only correct those errors cures." *Health Epigrams* – Dr. J.H. Tilden

Benefits eventually replace discomforts. They make fasting gratifying and well worth the effort.

Fasting clears the blood and the body of:

- Toxins, poisons, body wastes
- Chemicals, cigarettes, alcohol, caffeine, drug
- Addictions: drugs, chemicals, cigarettes, alcohol
- Allergens and their distressing symptoms

- Sugars, sweets, as well as any urges
- Cravings and dependence on sugars, drugs, etc.
- The body and the mind and the emotions
- Tensions, fears, fatigues and depressions
- Blood pressure and cholesterol

Sick, toxic cells are replaced by pure healthy ones.

Fasting revives and restores:

- Energies and enthusiasm
- Your morale and self image
- Spiritual and emotional awareness
- Tastes and desires
- Better living and eating habits

Fasting helps to restore the healthy functioning of...

- Damaged or sick organs and tissues
- Ulcers of the stomach, duodenum or skin
- Tired liver, heart, kidneys and pancreas
- Organs of detoxification
- Colitis, inflammations, infections of intestines
- Prostate problems, frequent urination and congestion
- Infections
- Discharges from female organs
- The causes of many diseases, as well as the disease themselves

Is one fast enough?

Can a body, even one that is in excellent health, in just a few days get rid of all the pollutant, toxins, wastes, excesses, poisons, drugs and chemicals that have accumulated in the system over many years – even most of a lifetime?

When, how often, can a fast be repeated?

Weekly, one-day fasts are a great way to maintain peak health. For one day a week, refrain from just eating a breakfast and lunch. Go from supper to supper, without food. Take only liquids, according to suggestions above.

Repeating longer fasts: four-to-10 days are recommended every three-to-six months. If symptoms indicate a lot of toxicity and really have a need to detoxify, fasting every six-to-eight weeks would be very much to one's benefit. Otherwise two-to-three short fasts each year is highly recommended.

After fasts there can be a problem

During the time no food enters the stomach, there is no stimulation of the saliva, stomach or pancreas glands. There is little or no secretion of their enzymes. During any or all fasts, it can be very helpful to supplement the needs of a body to catabolize all its wastes and dying cells with extra amounts of pancreatic enzymes. They are powerful detoxifiers.

If fasting has been only for a few days, glands will quickly return to secreting their normal amounts of enzymes. There is little likelihood of any digestive inadequacy. After very long fasts, the secretions take longer to return to their previous or normal levels.

As soon as you start back on foods, these enzymes have to be secreted in order to digest the foods you ingest. As stomach and pancreas that are lazy because of the fasting, won't do this right away. This is the reason why one must start back on food slowly and carefully. It invites the digestive organs to come to life again. As they do, one can return to eating their normal amounts of foods. Or, as an alternative, even before the digestion is able to work as it should, this problem can be resolved easily and readily by merely taking the enzymes in a supplement form. You may require hydrochloric acid, and stomach enzymes, as well as those of the pancreas.

Contra-indications to fasting

Unless there is an immediate urgent need to fast, there are times when fasting should not be undertaken, or if done, only after consulting with, and under the guidance of your holistic physician.

Contra-indications to fasting are...

- Nervous, physical, mental, emotional burnouts and exhaustion states, etc.
- Severe deficiency states.
- Serious stresses, distresses and traumas.
- Mental, physical or emotional overloads.
- Cancer, degenerative, chronic and other serious diseases. These do benefit greatly by fasting when done properly with the professional guidance.
- You have fasted. Now you are back to your normal life. Many of the toxic barriers to living have been emptied from your body and your life. Hopefully, life will now be a little bit more super normal.
- Part of the super-normal should be incorporating feasting into your life, after the fasting. The purpose of living is to live life to its peak – to live with enthusiasm, to live intensely – to really live everything that is in you.
- It would be good and valuable if you would include in the concepts of fasting the refraining from the cutting out and the eliminating from your life all the negativities, all the emotional and mental toxins and replace them with positive feasting – like the following.

Fasting from...	Feasting with...
Negative thoughts, attitudes	Positive thoughts, attitudes
Discontent, anger, resentment	Goodwill, caring, helping
Pessimism, sourness	Optimism, beauty, hope
Worry, anxiety, fears	Carefully thought-out living
Bitterness, hatreds, grudges	Forgiving, understanding
Work overloads	Light, pleasant burdens
Hostilities, getting even	Accepting, letting go
Self-pity, sorrowful feelings	The sunshine of serenity
Ego trips, selfishness	Joys – a part of caring
Stress excesses	Accepting life as it comes
Cheap, superficial pleasures	Soul-lifting experiences
Compromising self and needs	Total self-fulfillment
Suspicions, doubts, and skepticism	Trusting and believing
Gossip, petty talk, criticism	Purposeful silences
Crippling habits are thought	Uplifting ideal, goals
Wasting time, idle moments	Enthusiastic activities
Impatience, irritability	Patience, tolerance
Complaining, dissatisfaction	Appreciation, enjoying
Vulgar thoughts, words, acts	Gracefulness, respect
Disease-inducing lifestyle	Healing power of life, of God

Problems, difficulties,	Logic, realistic answers
Holding onto sorrows, hurts	Joys of living
Depressing, demoralizing facts	Uplifting ideas, ideals
Self-concern	Compassion for others
Complaining, fault-finding	Saying only good things
Thoughts of illness	What makes you feel good
Judging others	Giving others credit

Such elimination of negativities and allowing only positives can generate powerful positive benefits in our bodies and in our lives.

ALL fasting should always be a joyful experience.

You would like to get healthy, then try a fast.

When you feel how good it feels, you will be sorry you didn't try one a lot little earlier in your life.

Keep smiling – you are on the FAST track!

~~~~

CLEANSING PROGRAM

For those who are brave enough to try raw foods or want to transition to a raw food diet, this is an excellent starter diet. You must eat fresh vegetables and fruits and other raw plant foods. Your success with this program will depend on how closely you can follow it.
~~~~

1. Eat all vegetables and fruit cleaned and raw. MAKE SURE A VARIETY OF FOODS ARE EATEN. Have small amounts of different foods rather than a lot of one or two foods.

2. Drink liquids one half-hour before and one hour after a meal. Avoid drinking during meals. This means that you can have a small amount of liquid at these times or sips of liquid with your meal to wash it down.

3. Raw, unroasted and unsalted nuts, bean sprouts, and mild cooking spices (e.g. garlic used sparingly, basil, thyme, etc...) can be eaten. Avoid "hot and spicy" seasonings (e.g. table salt, curry, black pepper, hot peppers – but cayenne or red pepper may be used sparingly only if it does not bother your stomach).

4. Do not mix vegetables with fruit in the same meal because they can interfere with each other's digestion. Wait an hour or two between each. Generally, the order for food combining with this program and with regular meals is: firstly carbohydrates (starches such as breads, potatoes, carrots), followed by proteins (beans and grains, meats, fish, tofu), lastly fats (dairy products, oils, creamy foods). This order is suggested because it is related to the speed of digestion of each of these foods (i.e. carbohydrates break down first, while fatty foods are last). There are exceptions to the rule, generally and for individuals, but try this outline first.

5. Eat melons alone (watermelon, winter melon and cantaloupe).

6. NO sugar, candies, sweets, pastries, or packaged snacks. Avoid using self-administered medications.

7. Over the day, keep fluids (water, or vegetable and fruit juices mixed 50 percent with water) going through your body unless you have real problems with fluid retention. You do not need to force fluid down but pay attention to yourself and do not ignore your feelings of thirst. A juicer will give you real vegetable and fruit juice, and if used regularly it will be well worth the cost.

8. If any food gives you indigestion or discomfort, record it and let you clinician know. Do not eat those foods that cause problems for now.

Fruits:

Apples, apricots, bananas, blueberries, cherries, grapes, lemon, plums, pears, papayas, strawberry, watermelon, etc...

Coming off a Raw Food Diet

1. MOST IMPORTANTLY, DO NOT OVEREAT.

2. DO NOT SPLURGE ON "JUNK FOOD". EAT SENSIBLY.

3. Gradually eat more (of your usual) food, but follow the guidelines and your common sense. You may prefer to avoid some of your usual foods or to eat less of them (e.g. red meats). If you have any questions, ask your clinician.

Food Sensitivities

Food sensitivities can be related to allergies or other disturbances in your functioning. A simple way to monitor yourself to discover "disagreeable" food is described below.

For the first week or two, eat one new food per day. If you feel indigestion, headache, mood change, a flushed feeling over your face, or you feel uncomfortable after eating a food, avoid it for the time being as your body does not agree with it.

Gastrointestinal Detox Care: Keeping Intestines Clean, Keeping the Body Free of Toxins

We live in a poisoned, polluted world. A poisoned polluted world lives in us.

There are a multitude of hazards that threaten our health. Pollutants surround us, saturate us, threaten our health and undermine our integrity, our happiness, our abilities to think, feel and love. Pollutants threaten to undermine our inner world and ecology, as much as they affect and destroy our outer world and the ecology of Mother Nature.

There are too often repeated sayings regarding the intestines:

"Death begins in the colon." – Earl Irons. And...

"Ninety percent of all diseases start in the intestines."

Almost all the causes of our intestinal problems start in the digestive system, in the elementary track. It is not just the intestines that are at fault or affected. Up to 90 percent of all poisons and pollutants that affect our health are taken in by the mouth, then are normally or abnormally processed by our digestive system.

The first focus is on the word clean - get the intestines clean. To clean the intestines is simple. Take some laxatives, take five or ten flax or psyllium seeds, drink prune juice, take Bentonite or yucca, take an enema or a colonic. They all work well.

Keeping the intestines clean, and preventing the re-polluting of them, is a much more complex problem – a problem that requires a much more effective solution.

We need to master the art of keeping our intestines clean. Prevention of intestinal pollution means to bar access of toxins, abnormal foods, rotting and putrefying substances, chemicals, drugs and all forms of hazardous substances.

It is not possible to prevent or correct intestinal toxicity and keep it free of reoccurring poisons without knowing and understanding...

- What are toxins? What is toxicity?
- How do poisons work?
- Why and how are they toxic?
- Which substances are toxic?
- How toxic are they?
- Where do they come from?
- How to remedy and control them?

What are Poisons?

Poisons are substances that react with, damage and/or destroyed, where out and deplete enzymes without which organs cannot utilize proteins, minerals, trace minerals, starches (sugars) and oils nor are able to function. Without enzymes, we would starve. We would not sustain life for more than a few minutes.

The Webster dictionary states: "Any agent which introduced into an organism, may chemically produce any interests or deadly effect, or exert a baneful influence on, corrupt, preferred, and/or inhibit the activities of a catalyst." The key word is "catalyst".

But the definition does not tell us what the catalyst is. Without understanding catalysts we are still in the dark about the nature of a poison.

The catalysts of all biochemical reactions are enzymes.

Enzymes were briefly mentioned in the previous chapter, but here it's important to discuss it more deeply, especially since enzymes are critical to colon health.

It is not possible to appreciate the action and hazards of poisons without understanding enzymes: what they are, how they work in the body and what are their enemies that destroys them.

All enzymes are micro-molecules of protein. Many are combined with trace minerals.

Enzymes are created by the micros - the chromosomes of all cells. There are no other substances that have such power over life, that act, react, perform so many functions; create our life forces and so much of what we live by, as enzymes do.

The Nature of Enzymes

Enzymes are the doers, the operators, the workers that make possible all living and every conceivable function of our bodies, minds and emotions. They are the spark of life, and the powers that make possible everything in living: how we feel, how we think, use our muscles and moves, keep the heart going, maintain our body heat, digest foods, release life forces from foods and put them to work in our bodies in order to maintain biochemical balance and health.

There are possibly 500 million enzymes at work in our bodies. They are the carpenters which construct us. They are our demolition workers. They destroy and help eliminate all old, dead cells and cell debris.

Enzymes are body guards and health protectors. They are the life of our bodies, cells and organs. They are the forces which activate and try virtually every biochemical process that occurs in our bodies.

Our bodies obtain the raw materials from which enzymes are manufactured, from our digested food. These raw materials must be perfectly intact and available to the cells that need them. Our cells absorb the enzymes building material. They filter into the nuclei. There they are processed by Mike by chromosomes. They react to, combined with, neutralize and render harmless all abnormal and poisonous substances.

They should be no enzyme enemies in our bodies. Enzymes must not have been denatured or destroyed before they enter into our body.

Our Enzyme Factories

There is only one enzyme factory in our world: living cells - all cells. Every cell can create up to 200,000 enzymes. The chromosomes of all living cells of plants, animals, birds, fish and humans are nature's enzymes factories.

The amount of enzymes each plant cell manufactures is limited only by the amount of proteins and trace minerals it can obtain from the soil, air, and the energies they can obtain from the sun. The amount of enzymes in our body cells can manufacture depend on the amounts of quality proteins and trace minerals in the foods we eat and on their proper digestion, metabolism, and absorption.

Without enzymes life itself does not and cannot exist.

Unless one fully realizes the miraculous nature, roles and importance of enzymes, it is not possible to fully realize the disastrous effects that come from destroying them and/or not replenishing them according to our bodies needs. Anything that destroys enzymes undermines and threatens the functions, the structure and the very life of our bodies.

Enzyme Activities

Most chemical reactions in our body take place at high speeds. Enzymes are slow acting biochemicals. Acting alone, enzymes are not capable of acting at speeds required for living and by the demands of every cell and of every function of our bodies and minds. Enzymes need activators – accelerators. The activators and accelerators of enzymes are vitamins. This is the only role vitamins play in our bodies' activities. Vitamins alone, without their specific enzymes, are incapable of creating anything in the body that is conducive to living or a feeling. Enzymes and vitamins must always work together. They work as a team.

Vitamins could be compared to gas pedals in cars and enzymes to the motors. The motors do all the work. The gas pedals only help the motors to increase their speed.

However, even the enzymes and the vitamins working alone cannot fulfill all the needs or functions of living, and comply with and provide all the demands of our bodies' physiologies. They can function only as teams with other body biochemicals. They must and can work only, in association with specific proteins, minerals, trace minerals and oils.

Only with a thorough, in-depth knowledge of the structures and functions of cells can we understand and appreciate the tremendous role that enzymes play in our living, feeling and function. We need insights into "the world of the living cell". We need to understand how cells are created, how they function, what sustains and maintains them, what protects them from harm, what are their enemies and poisons.

Chemical, Drugs: Their Toxic Effects

Every chemical, every drug, every unnatural, dead, processed, refined substance destroy enzymes; uses them up and/or wears them out. Every tampering with natural substances, seized by man or chemistry, can only destroy. It can never improve. What man destroys are enzymes.

All chemicals and unnatural procedures denature and destroy the proteins and minerals which formed the structures, the membranes, the internal components of the cells (its protoplasm) and the chromosomes of the nuclei. Others will react chemically with one or more of the biochemicals in our body fluids and denature them.

A simple example illustrates this: the chemical and poisonous action of arsenic. Arsenic destroys the enzymes, which makes available and utilize (metabolize) food sugars and transform them into energy. Our living obtains a great deal of the life forces from this metabolism of sugars.

Our brains and the functioning of our minds require as much sugar and sugar energy as the rest of our whole body. They cannot function properly without generous supplies of whole sugars. A body depleted of this food is eventually depleted of life itself.

Arsenic has an affinity for, combines with, and destroys, a group of enzymes called phosphatases. Phosphatases are enzymes which react with phosphates and phosphorus – nutrients that are normally found in foods.

The metabolism of sugar molecules is responsible for the production of more than 90 percent of the energy derive from carbohydrates. Phosphatases breakdown sugar molecules. They split them into a simple minute size sugar micro-molecule. In processes similar to the creating of energy by atomic fission, each splitting of sugar molecules releases considerable amounts of energy.

Sugars that have not been processed by their enzymes, and whose phosphorus molecules have not undergone enzymes splitting, cannot be utilized by the body. Nor can our bodies obtain energies they require from that sugar. Without this energy, our brains, nerves, molecules and other organs cannot function. Our cells, our brains and our bodies die.

A simplified chart below shows how the breakdown processes of sugar takes place. It illustrates a biochemical fragmenting of a healthy food sugar. It also shows how the failure to properly process sugar leaves it in a chemical form incapable of functioning as a food or as a source of life, or energy. In essence, it becomes useless. Anything our bodies cannot use or metabolize becomes foreign, unwanted and toxic substances. In the case of sugar, this occurs by the mere absence of, or interference with, but one enzyme – a phosphatase.

This diagram also illustrates that there are three ways to prevent our bodies and cells from obtaining their normal energy supplies from sugar. This same failure to metabolize foods also applies to all other body substances.

- Process or refine the sugar before eating it. This takes out the enzymes before the sugar is ingested.
- Eat the whole natural food-form sugar (the whole complex of sugar, proteins, enzymes, vitamins and minerals), but add to this sugar-food a chemical, which destroys the enzyme.
- Allow chemicals to be present in our bodies which will bring about destruction of the sugar complex, as it normally exists in the whole natural foods.

Sugar enters the body →

It is first acted upon by enzymes of both saliva and the pancreas. It then passes through the following states:

Glucose-6-phosephate
--acted upon by a phosphatase

Fructose-6-phosphate
--acted upon by a phosphatase
Fructose-1,6-diphosphate
--acted upon by a phosphatase
Gyceraldehyde-3-phosphate

Phosphatases are catalysts that combine and react with and split off the phosphates. Phosphatases are denatured and destroyed by arsenic. Each stage of sugar breakdown is blocked.

--acted upon by a phosphatase
Phosphoglyceric Acid
--acted upon by a phosphatase
Phosphopyruvic Acid
--acted upon by a phosphatase

Pyruvic Acid→In absence of oxygen→→ Lactic Acid
Lactic Acid→Acetyl CoA
With oxygen → CO_2+H_2O

Lactic acid is a waste chemical that creates fatigue, sometimes referred to as a fatigue poison.

As the molecules are split, a great deal of energy is liberated. This sugar cycle is complete. Notice that phosphorus/phosphates form part of the sugar phases in six of the eight breakdown states, and that in each step, sugar disintegration is triggered by a phosphatase.

Any steps can be wiped out by the presence of arsenic (and/or other poisons). Sugars and all foods can be a source of our life's energies only when they can successfully pass through each step of their processing (metabolism), when the phosphatases are available to metabolize them. If in any one step one enzyme is missing or is destroyed or inhibited, the sugar processing is blocked at that point.

Whether the sugar enzymes required to metabolize and utilize the sugars have been destroyed, refined or processed out before they are eaten, or have been destroyed by a chemical or poison, the effects on the body are the same. Refined sugars and foods become unusable substances incapable of creating any fuel-form energy. They become toxic wastes. They use up and deplete small amounts of our body's reserves of the phosphatase enzymes.

Although sugar has been used here as an example, the same applies to all foods and to vitamins and minerals, and amino acid supplements.

All enzyme-depleted substances should be considered as toxic hazardous substances – as mild poisons.

Seven main chemical terrorists that destroy enzymes: chemicals and drugs, heat, oxygen, freezing, radiation and microwaves.

Foods are transformed into useless, life-depriving substances by any of the following:

- Refining, processing
- Chemical treatments by additives, preservatives, artificial colorings and flavors, etc.
- Staleness, prolonged contact with air oxidizes enzymes
- Overcooking, overeating and excessive high heat
- Microwaves, enzymes/protein fragmenting vibrations
- Radiation is the most powerful destroyer of enzymes.
- Food freezing. Thawing causes rupture of the cell membranes. The substances inside the cells contact the substances of a different acidity outside of the cells. They interact chemically and mutually destroy each other. Enzymes are also destroyed.

Classic examples of foodless foods:

Refined white flour, sugar, salt, industry-massacred cereals, canned foods, overcooked and junk foods, instant foods, synthetic and preserved foods and most fast foods.

Pasteurizing of foods means that all the enzymes in those foods have been destroyed by heat. A test to determine whether the pasteurizing milk (or food) is complete or not, measure the level of enzyme destruction. Pasteurization is when all enzymes are destroyed. *Do you Really Want to Drink that Milk?*

The Digestion Processes

Digestion starts in the mouth by the action of saliva. There are enzymes in the saliva, which are needed to break down sugars. A lack of those saliva enzymes result in faulty digestion of sugars.

A lack of saliva enzymes can result either from an inadequate secretion from the saliva glands or a failure to completely chew the foods. The action of the muscles of chewing squeezes the saliva glands and increases the flow of saliva from them.

Stage I: Food Digestibility

Foods must first be in a digestible state. Digestibility depends on the state of the foods. Foods in their original state are cells which contain self-digesting enzymes. These agents starts the processes of auto-digestion and render foods susceptible to be acted upon by digestive enzymes. The enzymes inherent in the food cells themselves, auto-digest up to 75 percent of their own cell components before our body's digestive enzymes are called into action.

If the food cell enzymes are destroyed by chemicals, radiation, oxygen or overcooking, those cells cannot decompose (auto-digest) themselves. Our bodies are not able to process or use those foods as nutrients. They are literally no longer foods.

There is a simple test to determine if foods still contain their cell enzymes. Leave a portion of a food on a shelf for few weeks: a piece of bread, a carrot, a potato or a fruit. If weeks or months later you see no change, no rotting or decomposition, the enzymes of those cells were destroyed.

Cell enzymes are still intact in fresh alive, natural foods, then join with the enzymes secreted by our stomach and pancreas. They are able to disintegrate and fragment food cells and transform them into molecule size substances small enough to filter through the intestinal walls and enter into our systems, and be transported to cells where they can be processed and used. This is the digestion.

If auto-digestion and digestive enzymes action do not bring the digestion process to its completion, foods rot or decompose in the intestines, just as they turn into compost when left in a field. They become soil and plant nutrients. But in the intestines they are toxic. These rotting, putrefying food substances create a swamp in the intestines. They intoxicate and poison the delicate cells of your intestinal villa and walls. They denature the cells and create changes which eventually result in cramps or disease – even serious disease: Colitis, Crohn's Disease, Appendicitis, Diverticulitis, etc.

Stage II: Mastication, Saliva Enzyme Saturation

We have been taught that the enzymes from our saliva glands, stomach and pancreas completely digest foods. This is only part of the truth and of the digestive process.

Chewing crushes the foods so that the saliva can penetrate into every molecule and their enzymes can chemically act on those molecules. Large food morsels that are not masticated, crushed and broken down into small particles cannot be thoroughly acted upon by the saliva, nor acted upon later by the digestive secretions of the pancreas. They will not be completed digested.

Stage III and IV: Digesting and Processing Foods

The action of enzymes of the stomach and intestines are discussed throughout these pages and in particular the final chapter, entitled *Gastrointestinal Care*.

Intestinal Poisons, Toxins, Pollutants

Ninety percent of all toxins and poisons that affect our bodies and pollute our intestines are those that are taken in by the mouth.

There are four main types, and sources of, intestinal pollution:

1. The failure of our body to properly digest all foods.
2. The excess intakes of wrong foods, dead foods, junk foods, synthetic foods, chemically treated and overcooked foods.
3. Cooking proteins. This promotes the release of protein molecules of the original meat or food before the digestive processes have had the chance to transform them into harmless and readily utilizable amino acid molecules. These foreign protein molecules have a different chemical nature and structure than those of the human body.

4. The ingestion of toxic substances, chemicals, drugs.
5. Constipation means stagnation of pollutants.

Abnormal, chemically isolated, processed proteins are also toxic. Any researcher who injected pure natural proteins into the bloodstream of an animal observed that they are capable of killing the animal. If absorbed into the bloodstream of humans, they can cause a severe allergic reaction, which can result in severe shock.

Fermenting Foods

Poorly digested sugar, starch and carbohydrate foods ferment.

Putrefying, Rotting Foods

Any failure of the stomach to secrete sufficient quantities of hydrochloric acid or stomach enzymes blocks the digestion of proteins.

Any failure of the pancreas to secrete all its enzymes in sufficient amounts blocks the transformation into utilizable substances of fats, oils, sugars, starches and proteins. The pancreatic enzymes are responsible for the final breakdown stage of all foods.

Undigested or incompletely digested proteins putrefy and give off a foul odor. Anything that is not utilizable by the body can, and should be, considered as a toxin or a poison. Abnormal, denatured and undigested proteins can be very toxic – toxic enough to contribute to cancer. The intestinal gas rising from protein putrefaction is as toxic as a mini dose of arsenic.

There are many sources of body pollution and toxicity besides abnormal and abnormally digested foods. There are 15 other categories of enzyme-depleting substances which overload our alimentary system with all kinds of abnormal and toxic wastes.

Most of us pollute our intestines with a number of toxic chemicals and wastes every day of our lives. We do this unknowingly and then we are surprised when we become ill.

Synthetic, Instant, Unnatural, Refined and Chemically-processed Foods

These include all unnatural foods, the imitation foods, soft drinks, artificial fruit drinks; radiated, canned, overcooked foods, the isolated, refined substances in which original natural states have been tampered with and denatured by man or chemicals.

In this age, dominated by chemistry and science, we have been conditioned to believe that man and science can, at will, disregard the nature of things, process and change, fragment and denature, chemically pervert, and still expect that the end product will not be in disharmony with the biochemical nature of our bodies.

Just breathing pure oxygen without its normal teammates and synergists that always come together in nature, illustrates this point. There is no element on earth that we need more than oxygen. Yet breathing this in a pure form, when the nitrogen and the other elements of air have been removed (except for short periods of time), is detrimental to our health.

There is little difference in doing this and extracting one single chemical substance like a vitamin, mineral or an amino acid from foods, putting them into a tablet form and claiming that they have the ability to improve the body or even heal. The same idea applies to every other substance that man has refined and from which have been extracted all the elements, which nature created to function as part of biochemical teams.

Our Body's Catabolic Wastes and Toxins

Several billion cells die in our bodies every day. Cells, in dying, are like cadavers. They disintegrate and break up into piles of worn-out, decaying, body-polluting, toxic molecules. Every molecule needs to be taken care of, broken down, neutralized, detoxified, and rendered harmless. If the waste products and debris of these food cells are not properly and completely handled and eliminated, they putrefy, ferment and/or rot exactly as do foods in our intestines, as described earlier. They would accumulate and overrun our bodies. They would eventually flood our systems and cause disease or death.

The only agents our bodies possess to do this are again our enzymes. Since all enzymes are specifically oriented, each to one job alone, the only enzymes with the abilities to breakdown dead cells molecules are the same enzymes that digest and disintegrate dead cell molecules of the foods we eat. All dead and abnormal cells are treated by our digestive enzymes in exactly the same way as they attack food orders or steaks coming into our stomachs.

Some of this mass disintegration of dead cell molecules will pass into the intestine to be eliminated. Incomplete enzyme processing will leave them, likely undigested foods, discussed above, to putrefy and rot, and increase intestinal toxicity.

Digestive enzymes, mixed with digested foods that pass through the intestinal walls during the chemical processes of digesting those enzymes, were not destroyed. Digestion constantly and literally takes place in every corner of our bodies. Together, they pass into the bloodstream and penetrate into every tissue and body fluid. They disintegrate and digest all sick, dying, devitalized, abnormal or foreign cells and abnormal body wastes and cell debris.

Food Chemicals and Additives

Three thousand or more hazardous chemical preservatives, colorings, bleaches, chemical food colorings, thickeners, thinners, emulsifiers have been added to our foods by our commercial food companies. At least thousands of them have been proven to contribute to the cause of cancer. Another thousand have never been tested. Tests have not been done to determine the nature or toxicity of substances created by the various reactions that take place between chemicals when they interact with each other and form new ones. Tests have not been done to detect what they do in our intestines.

Preservatives

The word "preservative" is a brilliant invention by the food industry. It misleads us to believe that they are added as food protectors and that they prevent foods from spoiling. They do. However, only by destroying the enzymes of those foods they act on. "Preservatives" are embalming fluids, which mummify what they touch. "Preserved" means the foods can no longer be digested or metabolized. It is impossible for our body to obtain nutrients and benefits it needs from those foods. They will only stagnate in our intestines as mummified substances. They are toxic.

Not to be lightly dismissed are the waxes applied onto many foods to make them shine and prevent their rotting. Foods are coated to cut off their contact with oxygen in the air. If not properly dissolved by hot water or other solutions, some of these waxes are known to favor and contribute to the onset of cancer.

Read labels. Read them on every item you purchase, be it grocery stores or health stores.

Even read the labels on products sold by health food stores and other health product dealers. If you are not familiar with the words on the labels, they are chemicals. Don't ever put anything into your body that has any chemicals added to it. Check them out! Find out what these chemicals are and what they do.

Dead Foods, Overcooked Foods, Fried Foods

Heat destroys food enzymes. Cooking foods at temperatures above 165°F, or longer than a few minutes, will kill all the enzymes in the food. The highest and most destructive heat is that of frying. High heats make oils turn rapidly rancid and toxic.

Food Fats, Fat Foods and Rancid Oils

Fats are the tissues in which animals store their body wastes and abnormal substances. Each morsel of fat we eat, puts into our bodies the toxins of the animals for which the fats came. They can be highly toxic.

Too often oils are considered as fat foods. Nutritionally, there is as much difference between fats and oils as there is between black and white.

Oils are essential to health. But when stale, overheated and stored on shelves for long periods of time, they become rancid. Fats and rancid oils, including the ordinary store-bought mayonnaises and salad dressings, and hydrogenated bought oils (the worst being margarine) are the most toxic of all foods – surpassed in toxicity only by drugs and chemicals.

Barbecuing is an excellent example of fat toxicity. The fats melt and drip into the charcoal flames. The chemistry of the fats is transformed by the burning coals into substances of greatly increased toxicity – a toxicity accepted by medical research as an important cause of cancer.

Eating one barbecued steak, hamburger or other fat meats, has the same toxic effects on the body as the smoking of 30 packages of cigarettes.

Radiated Foods

Radiation kills everything it touches. Radiation destroys foods as it does cancer cells or other normal cells. The whole world atmosphere is supersaturated with radiation. The radioactivity levels are now three times more the human tolerance levels. Everything you touch and eat is now at least slightly radiated. Industry is radiating more and more of our common foods. Neither we, nor our foods, can be free of it. Nor can we escape from being affected by it.

Microwaves and Microwaved Foods

The destructive power of microwaves is 500 times greater than that of high tension wires. Microwaves are a different form of radiation. The micro-waves are high frequency vibration which shake, shatter, separate and denature molecules of proteins. They do this to the proteins that form the membranes and the components of the cells of the microwaved foods. They do this to the proteins that go to make up enzymes.

Proteins that have been denatured cannot be digested or handled as they need to be. Our bodies do not have enzymes to process abnormal, denatured proteins. Body vitamins and minerals are rendered useless. Depriving cells of their protein-structural materials is conducive to the breakdown of membranes, chromosomes and other cell components. Denatured proteins are toxic, toxic enough to help turn healthy cells into cancer cells. One of the amino acids microwaves create (D-Proline) is a nerve poison. Russian scientists outlawed microwaves in 1976. (G. Lubec C. Wolf, B. Bartosch, the Landcet, 67677:1992 to 1993. December 1989.

The Scavenger Foods

All scavenger animals, birds or fish, such as pork, rabbits, jackals, shellfish, eels, vultures, fish without scales and other birds, and animals are toxic. Scavenger foods are not foods for man. They are not fit for human consumption. This is not because of the abnormal or garbage foods they scavenge and eat, but because the chemistry of their flesh is different to, foreign to, and incompatible with the biochemistry of the human body.

The results of 30 years devoted to research on white blood cells by Dr. Gruner, a maverick in nutrition-oriented pathologist from McGill University proved this. These cells are our blood scavengers. They literally gulp and consume, and help detoxify whatever poisons are free floating in the blood. In poisoned blood, they swell up like sponges.

People show white blood cell bloating after eating meals of pork and other scavenger animals. Eating scavenger foods dumps as many toxic substances into the blood as is normally present in those who have cancer. Cancer is a disease that overloads the blood with so many toxins that the white blood cells decrease 35 percent inside. This percentage indicates a high probability of cancer.

The scavenger foods were listed in the ancient books of *Deuteronomy* and *Leviticus*. They were forbidden to man.

Foods, Minerals and Acids

In order for plants to manufacture their full quota of enzymes and life-sustaining nutrients, they must obtain from the soil they grow in well over 100 minerals. Not to add all these to our soil is to create foods poorly capable of sustaining a long life.

For a majority of people, around 90 percent of their daily intake of foods is acid. They produce an acid effect on the body. This is three-to-four times more acid than the body needs or can tolerate. All foods, except fruits and vegetables, leave an acid residue in our bodies. These are mainly candies, sweets, refined grains, (breads, pastries, cakes, pies, cookies, etc.), most seafood, beans, meats, and eggs.

Fermented foods: cheeses, yogurt, beer, wines, vinegar foods, pickles are highly acid foods. The most acid of all foods are soft drinks.

Acid foods and increased levels of body acidity create energy. Energy becomes activity. Each bottle of soft drink puts into our intestines and bodies an amount of acid that, if completely absorbed and utilize, would maintain body acid levels for up to one month. Soft drinks are 10 to 100 times more acidic than the body can tolerate. Acid excesses over activate and eventually wear out and deplete enzyme reserves – just as poisons do.

Poisons, Chemicals, Drugs, Chlorines, Chemotherapy, Pleasure Drugs

We inherited a huge surplus of chemicals after the last world war. Tens of thousands of tons of chemicals, created for war use, were surplus leftovers. There was no way to dispose of them, so they dumped them into our soil, into our waters and into our foods. From some of those chemicals, they created pesticides.

Pesticides kill not only insects, but birds, fish and animals. Nobody born after 1945 and living in the standard conditions of our cities and civilization, has for one minute of their life, been free of chemicals and pollutants.

Chemicals destroy enzyme in our foods, as well as those in our intestines and body. They cause cancer.

The chemical companies dumped (still dump) chemicals into our rivers and lakes. Almost everything is now polluted: all air, water, soil, foods and drugs, us included. They created medical drugs, dumped chemicals into prescription pills. They created food additives, colorings, flavorings, thickeners, thinners and preservatives, and dumped them into our daily foods. By poisoning our foods, they help us so that we can die without any insect bite, and feed our stomachs with food (dead) with no insects or worms.

Pesticides and Chemical Fertilizers

Almost all commercial foods are grown using chemical fertilizers. Any chemical powerful enough to kill insects and pests, kill cells which make up foods. Chemical fertilizers kill worms in the soil. Worms are essential to the growth and health of plants and foods.

These powerful chemicals also destroy enzymes in the soil and in the roots of plants. They block plants from absorbing nutrients they need from the soil. Mixed in with the foods they saturate, they poison the cells of the walls of our intestines as they come in contact with them.

We are told to wash them off our foods by soaking them in a diluted vinegar solution. This only washes pesticides off the surface of the foods. While the foods are growing, rain falls, flushes pesticides off plants and into their soil. They seep into the plants. They filter up trunks of trees and go into the flesh of fruits. The foods become so saturated and poisoned, that they kill bugs or worms that are buried in their flesh.

Teeth Amalgams (Fillings)

Minute amounts of mercury constantly dissolve off of amalgams. They dissolve into saliva and pass into our intestines. Some get into the blood stream that flows in and around our teeth. Via the blood, it goes directly to our brain and pituitary gland.

Root Canals

When the canals of teeth get damaged enough that dentists insist they need root canals, they almost get infected. The infection inevitably infiltrates into thousands of microscopic canals and spread through the rest of the tooth.

Unless a person's general health and resistance to infection are on a very high level, the infection that saturates the tooth (or teeth) will gradually and steadily seep out of the tooth into the blood and into the rest of the body.

An infected body is never a healthy body. This infection can be a serious barrier to the body's abilities to heal itself of other diseases, especially serious degenerative ones.

Fluorides in Drinking Waters, Toothpastes

The mining and other industries have no place to dump their fluoride wastes. The industries created the scam of using knowledge that fluorides have a strong affinity for calcium. In combination with calcium, it makes the calcium harder. They push this point to persuade dentists to use it, claiming that it stops tooth decays. Not so. It only delays cavities. The bacteria and sugars, and other cavity-inducing factors keep working anyway. It just takes them longer to break down the tooth's enamel, but at what price?

Fluorides are some of the most powerful enzyme destroyers known to science. Fluoride is 15 times more poisonous than arsenic. They are used in research studies whenever enzymes are to be destroyed in order to test the differences between living substances with and without enzymes.

About 90 percent of our bigger cities in North America have been fluorinated. To drink more than four glasses of water or eat foods prepared with, or boiled in water that is chlorinated, such as tea, coffee, soups, is to absorb overdoses beyond our body's tolerance.

Tobacco

Tobacco contains at least 16 proven causes of cancer. Tobacco is a radioactive. The radioactivity comes from the potash with which most all tobacco fields are fertilized. Potash is a pure chemical form of potassium. It is not commonly known that such a pure, processed chemical of potassium is about 50 percent as radioactive as radium. (The tobacco industry knows this). It has been estimated that the poisonous effects of each cigarettes cut 20 minutes from our lives.

Prescription Drugs

Using drugs as therapies is based on the principle of infuriating the body, and thereby, activating all their powers against the effects of the drugs. As the body wars against these drugs, its fighting abilities react against the diseases at the same time. The end result is a healing, but at what price? A destruction of enzymes and body immunity, and weakening the body against future diseases.

Antibiotics (Anti=against, antagonistic to; bio=life)

Antibiotics are microbial "pesticides". They have about the same efficiency, toxicity and side effects in our bodies, as pesticides have on insects. They add to intestinal toxicity. They destroy the normal healthy bacteria that keeps our intestines functioning as they must.

Mental Toxins

There are two kinds of mental toxins: the stimulators and the depressors.

Angers, resentments, anxieties, fears, worries, hatreds, self-hatreds are mind lashing toxins. They stimulate and whip the nervous system into a frenzy. They create stress, tension and uptightness. They cause muscles to tighten and tense up and blood vessels to contract. This decreases the flow of blood throughout our bodies.

Constant tenseness and toxicity contract muscles of the intestines. They become spastic. Constipation follows. Toxic substances in the bowels stagnate. They filter through the intestinal wall and passes into the body, and increase body toxicity.

Negative attitudes, grief, loss of hope, low self-image, depression, repression, low morale, guilt, and co-dependencies (dependencies on approval of others), are mind deadening toxins. These mental states slow down the brain and the whole nervous system. They slow down the blood circulation and decrease the nutrient, and oxygen supplies to all our organs. They slow down, depress and deactivate the nerves of the whole digestive track so that they cannot effectively function.

Both nerves and poor circulation affect the stomach, pancreas, intestines and colon. Sluggish nerves cause sluggish bowel elimination of the toxins and poisons that are stagnating in the colon.

Recognizing Toxins and Toxicity

This is done by....

- Evaluating how the body reacts to toxins.
- The diseases and breakdowns of body organs that result from excess toxin and poisons.
- Experiences of illnesses listed in the previous pages.
- A careful diagnostic history and physical examination, together with toxicological laboratory tests, such as blood, and urine, hair and feces.
- A "detective" type history and health evaluation that determines contact with, and ingestion of, pollutants.
- Observing the characteristics of the bowel movements. The pages and chart at the end of this book tell you what to look for and what each change means. It offers guidelines for figuring out all that is required for complete control of digestion and intestinal toxicity.

- The presence of a thick clear fluid (mucus) mixed in with BMs or floating on the toilet water. Mucus in stools indicates the presence of poison.
- Mucus is secreted by the cells of the intestines. Its role is to dilute toxins in the fecal matter which, not having been eliminated, contact the intestinal wall and its muscles and intoxicate or poison them. Mucus normally coats the intestine walls as a means of protecting itself against all irritation and toxicity.

Deleterious Effects of Body and Intestinal Pollutants

Constipation

Intestinal slow-down and sluggishness caused by stagnating wastes and pollutants is constipation. The constipated colon is a holding tank of body wastes and debris. When saturated with toxic substances and poisons, it becomes a cesspool. Poisons filter into the body, pass into the blood and create body toxicity.

Shorter Lives

Each poison that destroys an enzyme destroys a few minutes, sometimes a few hours of our life span.

Every time dead foods are allowed into our bodies, we add a little death into our lives. The lifespan of our years is roughly inversely proportional to the amount of toxic substances we allow in our bodies and retain in our intestines.

Mental – Nervous Diseases

Our brain and nervous system usually suffer first. Whatever gets into our bloodstream, goes directly to our brain. The brain and nerves are more sensitive and susceptible to poisons than other organs. Poisons and toxins either suppress our brain and nerve functions or over activate, over stimulate and whip the nerves until fatigued.

Brain/nervous oppression is experienced as headaches, migraines, dullness, fatigue, lassitude, discouragement, depression, melancholy, a foggy mind, sluggish thinking and mental processes, poor memory, lowered IQ and creativity; loss of our joys of living.

Overstimulation and whipping nerves, and brain causes neuritis, neuralgias, irritability, insomnia; agitated sleep, paralysis, twitching of any or various parts of our body.

Physical Ailments

Physical ailments of the blood vessels, loaded with their toxic blood, affect and afflict every organ.

Heart diseases

"There are a few phases of cardiovascular trouble (heart and blood vessels) with which a disorder of some part of the elementary tract is not causatively associated."- Dr. W. Bezley

Tuberculosis

TB is the result of intestinal intoxication. It is not possible for it to obtain a foothold in the lungs or in other organs, except that the lungs or organs were affected and polluted, and became fertile fields for fostering the growth of bacteria by the presence of toxins and wastes in their tissues, overflowing from the stagnating intestinal toxins.

These toxins develop first in the stomach. TB patients do not secrete sufficient amount of hydrochloric acid to either digest their foods (or thus keep their weight up), to disintegrate the TB disease. These bacteria are most sensitive to acids. They are sometimes called "acid-fast", meaning they are immobilized and neutralized by stomach hydrochloric acid.

Infections

Most bacteria are not toxic. By nature they are not our enemies as we have been taught to believe. In their natural state, they are our friends. They are micro-capsules of enzymes. Their chemistry originates from chromosomes. The bacterial makeup of bacteria is similar to both chromosomes and enzymes. Bacteria and viruses react with and absorb the toxins and poisons of their environment, and live on the substances they swim in. Diseased bacteria continue to multiply in proportion to the amounts of toxins they feed on. Only by keeping the body and intestinal environment clean and free of toxins can we keep them free from harmful bacteria.

Only bacteria that have been poisoned by passing through toxic and polluted inner body environment cause infectious type diseases. But they do this only after being poisoned by the poisons, which were the original and real disease. They become harmful and hazardous to health, only secondarily. Disease-causing bacteria are created by disease rather than the *cause* of the disease.

Immunity Breakdown

Loss of body resistance to disease leaves us prone to cancer, AIDS and other degenerative diseases.

Skin Problems

Buildups of skin toxins lead to skin problems and diseases. All skin diseases involve some weakening of the skin tissues from deficiencies and attacks on the skin by the poisons being eliminated through their pores. These lead to eczema, psoriasis, acne, herpes, dermatitis, lupus and cellulite.

Allergies

Allergies are manifestations of deficiencies, especially of the digestive enzymes –also those of the antihistamine-type enzymes, which is one of its normal functions the liver creates.

Obesity, Overweight

Body fat is the body's way of storing excesses of abnormal substances – substances that the body can't use – substances, which if left to float freely through our tissues, would clog up blood circulation and denature our body fluids – substances which could be harmful to our health. The body also extracts out of the blood and store away toxic chemicals and drugs.

Fibroids, PMS, Painful Periods

"Auto-intoxication plays a large part of disease in the development of female genitourinary apparatus, that they may be regarded by the gynecologist as a product of an intestinal stasis." - Dr. Lane

Pain

The first and most important, and most widespread effects of body poisons is pain. Ninety five percent of all pain is caused by the action on nerve endings of abnormal chemicals or poisons. The role of nerves is to sense the presence of abnormalities, chemicals, pressures and temperature changes. Nerves send signals to the brain, notifying it of these abnormalities. The brain activates defense or protective mechanisms to control or manage the abnormalities.

Some poisons, when in excess, can cause pains so severe that even morphine won't relieve them. There is so much pain in cancer, because the toxins are virulent and the amounts of poisons are high – more than in almost any other disease.

Intestinal cramps and pains result from stagnating poisons afflicting the nerves of the intestines. They have to be eliminated effectively and quickly. This is what diarrhea is all about. Cramps are forceful contractions of the intestinal muscles attempting to squeeze out and eliminate excess irritants and toxic substances.

Detoxification can relieve toxin-caused pain. When one completely eradicates all the poisons from the body, pain leaves. Few cancer patients, even terminal cases, experience more than minimal pain when their bodies are completely detoxified.

Allowing entry into our bodies, and stagnation of even small amounts of toxic substances, is an abuse to our health. It should never be tolerated.

Cancer

Poisons destroy normal cells and transfer them into toxic, wild growing cancer cells and tumors.

Cancer tumors indicate extreme and prolonged stagnating body toxicity, most of which is absorbed from the intestines. Cancer cells, like fat cells, have lost their normal functions. They have become storage cells for poisons. Tumors are masses of those poisons-storing cells. They are garbage pails. They take and absorb out of our tissues toxic substances, which endangers the very life of our organs and body. As such, tumors perform a valuable and even lifesaving role. They become our friends – not our enemies. It is the poisons that cause them, which are our enemies. Only occasionally, when they press on nerves or cause compression on organs, do they become harmful or life-threatening.

The storage cells can grow at a speed fast enough to absorb any excesses that need to be taken out of the body circulation. It is extremely difficult for cancer patients to get better, as long as their bodies' poisons continue to feed the tumors.

Those that will remain free of these dread diseases will be those who learn how to avoid chemicals and pollutants, and take the precautions of clearing their systems and intestines of all stagnating toxins.

High Blood Pressure

Toxins that filter through the intestinal wall pass into our blood stream. The blood vessels carry them directly to the liver. They overload our liver. Livers are like sponges. The toxins plug up and block the liver porosity. The blood that keeps pouring into our livers from every square inch of our bodies cannot get through. The volume builds up in all the blood vessels. This becomes high blood pressure.

All body poisons, toxins, wastes, chemicals and pollutants also affect muscles, joints, bones and ligaments. They create a weakness, fatigue, burnout, exhaustion and diseases.

The point to be made in listing all of the above diseases is that all of them could have been avoided by keeping our bodies and our bowels free of poisons, and pollutants.

Why do we not all feel serious disease and the effects of our poisons and pollutants?

The devastating effects of constant body toxicity may sometimes, not be felt for a long time. Those living close to nature or pollution free areas may still maintain sufficiently resistance to disease and poisons to escape the effects of chemicals they contact or ingest. As long as there are sufficient reserves of enzymes, we have little or no awareness of illness or toxicity. The power of cells to create self-protecting enzymes is amazing. It can take up to four generations to deplete them.

As long as we have plentiful enzymes, our bodies succeed in breaking down all the chemicals, poisons and pollutants.

As long as we keep nourishing our bodies with the protein and trace mineral elements needed to replenish our resources of enzymes, our cells will keep building them as fast as they get destroyed by their contact with poisons.

False Sense of Security and Health

Living life, which seems to be normal and free of disease, deceives us into believing that we are healthy, and therefore, does not harbor harmful amounts of toxins. However, no one living in civilization is free of toxicity. Nor do any of us know how much toxicity and poisons are stored away in our organs and tissues, and how much of them are putting our life at risk until we have undertaken an intense detoxification program and feel the differences of body, mind and emotions when freed from our slavery to the effects of those harmful pollutants.

Re-polluting our bodies exhausts our cells and tissues, and depletes them of disease-resisting enzymes. We get to a point where we can no longer create and replace the enzymes we need. When these enzyme reserves are run down, and are no longer adequately effective, we enter into states of distress we call disease. This can happen gradually, without any awareness on our part.

Advice for Healthy Intestines

One of the most important approaches to health is complete, thorough cleansing of the colon. This can be health saving and lifesaving. Be good to your intestines. Appreciate and care for it. Keep it clean and free of pollutants. Always have as many BM eliminations as the number of meals you eat. If toxic for a long time, there should be more BM movements than meals in order to catch up with the years of backlog.

Intestinal Cleaners

The most effective are bentonite, flax or psyllium seeds. Yucca or black radish herbs greatly add to the efficiency of elimination. When toxic, sick or constipated, use one or all of them on a regular basis.

Liver Cleansers

Several herbs are known to provide the liver substantial amounts of enzymes. They increase the liver's ability to detoxify, neutralize and eliminate the huge amounts of body toxins livers have to handle every day of our lives. Especially of value supporting the work of our livers perform in these ways are: dandelion roots, milk thistle and beet juice concentrates, as well as some of the following cleansers.

Bile Detoxifier

Bile is a toxin solvent. It is manufactured by our livers. Our livers dump their toxins into the bile. The bile carries these toxins directly to the intestines for elimination. At the same time, bile stimulates the muscles of the colon and speeds up the contractions and their elimination of fecal matter. It can work wonders as a pain reliever.

Fibrous Foods

All crisp foods, and especially bran, are rich in fiber. These should be used in generous amounts. Use a generous serving of salads and crisp, raw foods, like carrots, nuts, coconut and apples. Pour bran onto cereals, into soups, and onto salads.

Never use the commercial dry boxed cereals. Never use *All Bran* or processed bran substitutes. They irritate the colon.

Soft, mushy, overcooked or overheated foods - avoid them.

Oils

Use generous quantities of high quality oils. Oils are an important part of our body's resistance to chemicals and pollutants. Oils coat the lining of the intestines and block contact of toxins with the cells that make up the inner skin and the lining of the intestines. Oils pass into the body and coat every cell. This coating protects the cell from the onslaughts of body pollutants.

Lemon Juice

Mix one to two teaspoons of freshly squeezed lemon juice with a teaspoon of honey in a glass of warm spring or demineralized water. Upon rising in the morning, prepare yourself a delicious glass of warm lemonade. It mildly soothes and activates the intestines' flushing action.

Pineapple, prunes, papaya or fresh grapefruit, melon, watermelon, or their juices are very helpful in similar ways.

Fenugreek Tea is excellent for eliminating toxins.

Use when mucus is noted in the fecal matter. If you find the flavor is not pleasing, add a little lemon juice or a pinch of ordinary tea, or a teaspoon of unpasteurized honey.

Warm Peppermint or Chamomile Tea

These soothe the nerves, relax the stomach and intestines, and improve digestion. They are excellent taken between meals and/or after meals.

Exercise

The body needs much more oxygen than it needs foods. Our bodies need and use up to 150 pounds of oxygen a day compared to two to three pounds of food we normally eat. Bodies obtained this oxygen by muscle activity, which aids the heart and intensifies the flow of blood. It gets the blood flowing more abundantly, bringing more oxygen to tissues, including the muscles of the intestines and colon.

Alternating muscle contractions and expansions of exercise act as a pump on all our lymphatic vessels. These are the "sewer pipes" that drain toxins and wastes from every cell in our bodies and flush them into our livers for detoxification.

Exercise also activates the muscles of the intestines and promotes intestinal flushing.

Herbal Laxatives

When ill, no detoxifying is adequate unless every day, a greater quantity of body wastes, toxins and poisons are eliminated than consuming food. If there are less bowel movements than meals, start with a simple remedy: an herbal laxative of Senna, Cascara or Yucca. Some are strong and some are weak. You may have to use a "trial and error" approach to find the one that provides the best elimination without causing diarrhea or cramps.

Enemas

Enemas are intestinal flushes. They wash out effectively, and without pain, the toxic residues stagnating in the colon.

Enemas are to be used whenever your body...

- Fails to eliminate all its daily toxins
- Feels distresses, discomforts, and or (dis)ease
- Is experiencing reactions to the effects of good healing therapies, healing crisis

Directions: to be read carefully

From your drugstore, purchase a quart (or liter) sized enema bag. This is a hot water bottle with a small tube attached, plus a nozzle for inserting in your rectum.

Fill the enema bag with 1 L or 1 Qt of de-chlorinated water. The chlorine of tap water is toxic. It combines with matter in the bowels and forms chloroform. To de-chlorinate water requires only that you pour tap water into a container and let it stand on your counter for at least 24 hours. The chlorine evaporates.
Water that is demineralized or distilled can absorb more toxic substances than water still saturated with its minerals.

Enema water should be heated to your body temperature. According to your needs, and to provide other benefits, some herbs, teas or coffee can be added. The amounts used would be similar to those used in preparing a beverage to drink.

- If you experience, or your enemas cause irritation, spasms or cramps, add chamomile, peppermint, catnip tea or Aloe Vera juice.
- If mucus are seen in the stools, add Fenugreek tea.
- If debilitated and seriously ill, add wheatgrass juice or powder.

If very toxic add:

- Two tablespoons of bentonite mixed with psyllium seed powder.
- A tablespoon of Yucca herbs. Both of these bind with and carry out huge amounts of toxins from the intestines. The Yucca is soothing and healing to the irritated intestinal wall.
- If in real pain, or distressed use coffee enemas.

The Coffee Enema

This is a crisis detoxifier – an emergency bowel eliminator and a liver and body detoxifier. The caffeine in coffee is a strong stimulant. Caffeine taken by the rectum acts differently than when it is taken by mouth. It passes through the intestines and into blood vessels that carry it directly to the liver. The liver and intestines are sluggish when toxic. Caffeine stimulates and activates the liver and accelerates the flushing out of toxins from it. Coffee opens the bile ducts and increases the flow of bile.

Do not use coffee enemas daily or for long periods of time. Use only for one to a few days – not regularly. Use only as needed. Too much stimulation can tire out your liver and colon.

Preparing Coffee Enemas

- Use only fresh ground, lightly roasted coffee beans.
- Never use instant, stale or decaffeinated coffee.
- Store the coffee grounds that are not for immediate use in a freezer. Coffee beans contain oils, which once grounded, turn rancid. Rancid oils are toxic, even causes cancer.
- Prepare the coffee the same way as for drinking. Use a filter drip or a percolator or let boil for three minutes and simmer for 20 minutes more. Strain it.
- Never boil in aluminum pots, tea kettles or electric kettles. The heating elements of the latter are pipes of copper. These metals are irritating and toxic.

- It is best to prepare the coffee enema fresh each time. However, several quarts can be prepared ahead of time and stored in the refrigerator.
- Add two to three tablespoons of coffee grounds per quart. If you are sensitive or jittery, use a lesser amount. If well tolerated, and if or when severely ill or toxic, use greater amounts.

Directions for taking the coffee enemas

- Be comfortable. Relax as much as you are able. Relaxing allows the intestines to loosen up, to fill up and to eliminate better.
- Lubricate the nozzle with oil. Use a vegetable oil, KY Jelly or an ordinary ointment. (Never use Vaseline. It is a petroleum product.)
- Use nozzles calibrated at sizes 24 to 32. These are available from drugstores.
- Insert the nozzle as far in and as high as you can comfortably. Do this slowly with the rotating motion. This avoids kinking inside the colon. Kinking can occur from too rapid or too forceful insertion of the tube. If the bag does not empty freely and steadily, your enema tube may be folded on to itself (kinked). Pull it straight.
- Suspend the enema bag so that its lower edge is about one-to-one-half feet above your body. The height controls the speed of the water entering the colon. If the bag or container is too high, the solution runs into the colon too fast; if too slow, the flow is slow. It should take several minutes for the bag to empty the fluid into your body. The fluid's inflow should be comfortable. If it is too fast, you may feel cramps or stomach discomfort. If cramps start, slow the flow, by pinching or closing the enema tube. Then lower the bag. Wait until the cramps subside. Start again.
- Lie on the floor on a bath rug or on a large towel. Lie near the toilet. Lie on your left side or on your back. For some people, it is easier to get up (after taking their enema) from

their back rather than from the side. Or, be on your knees with the top of your chest touching the floor, your buttocks as high as possible. The latter position gives the added advantage of gravity favoring the flow of water down deep and far into the colon.

- Before defecating, remove the nozzle. Then lie on your left side for three to five minutes. Roll slowly onto your stomach. If you sense any discomfort in your abdomen, roll again onto your back. Stay in this position for another three to five minutes, then roll onto your right side for another three to five minutes. Total time is 10 to 15 minutes, if there is no serious discomfort. Eliminate what you have retained.
- If you find it difficult to retain the enema fluid inside for the full 10 to 15 minutes, get up and eliminate.

NOTE: If your enema is not thoroughly evacuated, take a second one 20 to 30 minutes later. This should bring the complete elimination of both.

Oil Retention Enemas

When other enemas don't eliminate enough, and/or when the bowels or rectum are sore or inflamed, use oil enemas.

- From a drug store, purchase a baby (one-cup capacity) enema syringe
- Use only good food quality oil, like sunflower, olive or soya oil. Add a teaspoon of freshly squeezed lemon juice to the oil.
- Warm the oil/lemon mixture to your body temperature. The oil lubricates the nozzle as you aspirate. Insert the nozzle into the rectum. Squeeze. Hold oil inside overnight. Have your normal bowel movements in the morning.
- Use these oil-retention enemas along with the ordinary enemas. It is suggested to use this type of enema every other evening. Use them after taking the evening enemas or after having your bowel movements.

If seriously ill, or afflicted with a degenerative disease, instead of the enemas, use colonics.

Colonics

A colonic is a glorified enema, an easier way of effectively cleaning out the higher regions of the colon. These are not always well reached or well cleaned out by enemas. Colonics require special equipment that has been designed to make this possible. They are called “colema boards.” They are not available in drugstores or from most health equipment outlets. They have to be ordered or given by a holistic practitioner.

Before using the colema boards, it is advisable to first take one or two colonic treatments from a professional colonic therapist. It is good training in learning how to take them. It will make you feel comfortable with what to expect, how it feels and how it works.

The number of enemas to be taken

Pain will not be relieved until you have sufficiently emptied the body of toxins or poisons, which are causing the pain. In crisis or severe pain states, it may be necessary to take a coffee enema every half hour until relief is experienced.

Take the minimum number of enemas that are needed for complete pain relief. The number of enemas you may need depends upon the severity of pain or disease. If the pain is severe or unbearable, you may require many – even many in a day.

You may feel little or no change or relief from one enema to the next, until the poisons are gone. At one point, the next enema will bring quick relief. This could happen after your fifth, 10th or 14th enema, or more. The relief feels a little like the sun coming out from behind a cloud.

As soon as this relief is sensed, the coffee enemas should be stopped. Take them again only when needed to relieve a reoccurrence of serious pain or toxic distress. Otherwise, when you need an enema take the gentler kinds suggested and described above.

The Advantages of Colonics

In serious, degenerative and toxic conditions, this is the most desirable form of detoxification. Up to five quarts of water are used to flush the intestines. This dislodges and flushes out much more fecal matter, debris and toxins than do the enemas or laxatives. The water works higher, digs deeper and right through to the upper regions of the colon. It works until everything is cleaned.

The Colon Purges

These are methods for radically and rapidly detoxifying the intestines, the liver and the body when you are very toxic.

The Epson Salts Purge

Upon rising, drink a half glass of water in which a tablespoon full of Epson salts has been dissolved.

The Purge Punch

Freshly squeeze six fresh lemons, 12 oranges and six grapefruits. Make the juices of these in a gallon jar. Fill with (demineralized) distilled water.

Drink a glass of this punch every hour (during the daytime), until the gallon is finished, or as much as you can. It is most effective if taken over a period of two days. If you are too weak, or taking the juices upset you strongly, purge yourself for only one day.

There are advantages to repeat purges every four weeks, especially when seriously ill, seriously toxic or your liver has been overloaded and congested for a long time. In such conditions, it should be repeated every four weeks.

NOTE: After purges, you may experience uncomfortable sensations, nausea, headaches, cramps and/or dizziness – feelings like a hangover. This result is from the sudden dumping of an abundant amount of poisons (that have accumulated and stagnated in your body over many years), from the tissues in which they were stored in the bloodstream. This dumping can be a shock to your system.

The reactions and sensations are temporary. They will disappear once the poisons are eliminated from your body.

Caution: Body detoxification can be too intense or too rapid

An effective therapy will sometimes breakdown more of the body's natural storehouses of wastes, debris's and toxins than the organs of detoxification and elimination can handle. The flushed out poisons pour back into the blood. They may flood the tissues. They can re-poison and harm the body the same as if you were to take those poisons by mouth for the first time.

Avoid as much as possible all the toxins, chemicals and poisons described in the previous pages. Obviously, in order to be able to avoid them all, you would have to leave civilization and go and live close to nature or in a wilderness. Doing your best usually suffices.

Don't focus your attention and fears on viruses, bacteria or on tumors and pain.

Remember: bacteria, viruses and infections are not to the boogiemen enemies of health. Bacteria are not evil. They are scavengers of body poisons.

` ` `

Nature creates no evil. Nature allows no evil to survive in us.

We sponsor, indulge in, and harbor the evils and allow them to affect our lives and our bodies.

Make a date with life every morning when you get up and celebrate that date with intense living.

Rejoice and live

Implement solutions

To your body pollutions or end in dissolution

Parasite – Worm Control

All parasites and worms are cells. Parasites are single cell infesters. Worms are multiple cell organisms. They are made up of cells constructed from proteins, just like human cells or the cells of animals and plants.

Parasites' cells and their physiology are different from human cells, and those of the individual they are infesting. Because of differences in their biochemistry, they are foreign to our bodies, irritating and detrimental to human physiology. By their nature, no living creature or organism, bacteria, virus or fungus is harmful, evil or destructive in itself.

Bacteria and parasites flourish in our bodies when they find and come in contact with a plentiful supply of sick, rotting and toxic organic substances. They live on these. They digest them and break them down. In doing so, they preserve and protect the body's cells and tissues from being affected by them. They do not and cannot attack or harm anything that is normal and healthy in our bodies.

They act as scavengers and destroyers of any and all substances which are abnormal, irritating, or toxic, to our body's blueprint. They secrete enzymes which disintegrate sick and dying, deficient, toxic or rotting cells and tissues. They transform abnormal, toxic and dead substances into soil food – into compost. By doing so, they restore nutrients to the soil and perpetuate the cycle of life.

The key point in dealing with all scavenger organisms, be they visible or microscopic in size, is that they cannot survive without their specific, nutrient needs. Their nutrients are always and only body wastes and debris, and the debris of sick, toxic, foreign and/or abnormal cells, or cells which have been damaged and are dying. They cannot live in a human body, unless toxicity and sickness is already in that human body. They live on sickness. Their role is to prevent, not cause sickness.

Parasites and worms cannot survive in an organism, an environment or a body which is highly saturated with all their normal needs of trace minerals. Trace elements are foreign to the makeup of all lower forms of beings like insects, worms and parasites. These vermin cannot digest, utilize or tolerate trace mineral concentrations. They are repulsed by them.

Eradicating Worms and Parasites

Parasites and worms can be drugged and killed just like any other form of living organism or cell. However, any drug (vermifuge-worm medicine) toxic enough to kill parasites or worms, will be toxic enough to kill human cells. All drug treatments of parasite and worms are toxic and hazardous to the health of who takes them.

Therapies more effective than drugs

First, restore your health. Follow whatever regime is required to provide your body with every required nutrient.

Correct all deficiencies. Eliminate all toxic accumulations, foreign substances; all substances that are not utilized by your body, and that are in excess of the body's needs.

Carefully rid your body of all causes of degenerative processes or diseases.

Start parasite purging by cleaning out the bowels with purging doses of herbal (nondrug and non-toxic) laxatives or good enemas. Eliminate excesses of fecal matter and of toxic residues in the intestines. These measures alone can successfully and effectively flush out parasites, or most of them.

Supersaturate the body, in particular the intestinal track with high levels of parasite-repulsing minerals.

- Each morning, upon rising, drink one glass of spring water with one teaspoonful of sea salt added to it.
- Use mineral rich liquid and herbal flushes.
- Take fresh garlic cloves in fresh foods. These are very repulsive to worms. Add parsley to eliminate the bad breath odor after eating the garlic.

- Generously spice foods with kelp, dulse, cayenne pepper and/or sea salt.
- Sage: Take one teaspoon with honey, one hour before eating, three times a day, for three days.

Use generous portions of foods, which interfere with worm activity and vitality. These are:

- Ground pumpkin seeds, onions, chamomile tea, asparagus, apricots, pomegranates, wheat germ oil (absolutely fresh only).
- Wheat germ oil pearls (or Cerol - Standard process). Take six to 10 pearls daily for at least three weeks. The oil coating on the intestinal wall, and on the parasites themselves, interfere with their abilities to contact and use the oxygen and the substances or toxins in that environment.
- It is preferable to take the oil concentrates on an empty stomach so that they can contact and act directly on foreign organisms stagnating in the intestines.

ALL proteins are readily digestible, be they proteins of parasites, worms and vegetable, or meat proteins. As an example, a piece of steak in the stomach takes only a few minutes to be reduced into totally digested liquid substance. A body's digestive enzymes disintegrate them. Any digestive enzyme can help. Normally, a three-week program containing many or most of the above can eradicate parasites, worms, pinworms, etc., from anybody.

Use the above suggested approaches daily for one week. Take immediately upon rising or midway through the afternoons. Stop for one week. Repeat for one week.

In the case of re-infestation, it will be necessary to find and eradicate the source of contact with parasites.

- Restore general health.
- Detoxify more intensely, for a longer time.
- Repeat the above program until well.

Evaluating digestive deficiency: a symptom survey and questionnaire stomach enzymes/HCL in adequacy symptoms

I burp right after meals__

Stomach burns after meals__

I have a poor appetite__

Appetite has always been poor__

Difficulties digesting meats and raw vegetables__

Stomach burning relieved by taking milk, acids and foods__

I sometimes get the hiccups after meals__

I often get as sour/acid taste in my mouth after meals__

I feel full and bloated within one to two hours after meals__

Sometimes I get nauseated; I may feel like vomiting__

I get a foggy heavy head and fatigue after meals__

Symptoms of inadequate pancreas enzymes

Abdominal cramps __ Stomach burning__

Stomach fullness__ Heaviness after meals__

Abdominal discomfort __ Digestive problems__

Fatigue after meals__ Mucus in throat__

Intolerance to fats__ Sugar intolerance__

I pass lots of gas__ Gas has no odor__

Gas has a foul odor__ Cramps pains below the naval__

Can only eat small meals__

Severe cramps/pains below midrib ribs five to six hours after food__

Belch, burp, low abdomen rumbling two to four hours after meals__

Use the symptoms to guide you in the choice of the types of digestive enzymes you may need. The more answers in either sections above, the more you may need enzymes of that type.

Abdominal Bowel Movement Characteristics

I have less number of bowel movements than meals I have eaten__

I have to force, it takes time to pass BMs__

Passing BMs is painful; rectum is tender__

There are spots of blood on toilet paper__

There is some blood in stools__

I pass only small amounts of fecal matter__

BMs are poorly formed; fragmented bits and trunks__

BMs are soft, mushy, not formed or diarrhea__

Stools are hard and dry, difficult to pass__

BMs are long, pencil thin, or like a rope__

Stools have many holes, empty spots__

Stools vary from firm to soft, well formed to mushy__

BMs are stringy; they show lots of fibers__

Stool chunks float near/on surface of toilet water__

Color of BMs is pale brown, orange, grey or chalky__

Seeds, corn, nuts, skins, show up in bowel movements/toilet__

BMs undigested food particles__

As long as there are any of the above abnormalities, observations should be made daily. What appears should be written into a report. This report should be presented to your holistic physician.

Testing for Constipation

What you see in the bowel movements is the result of your digestion. Normal bowel movements equal normal digestion.

Swallow, don't chew a handful of nuts or corn that is raw, frozen or barely cooked. Note the time of the meal when these were taken. __a.m./p.m.

Check bowel movements regularly. Note the times when the corn kernels or nut fragments appear. The number of hours they appear after swallowing is__

Improvement in symptoms and BM characteristics is a measure of the improvements in your digestion and general body health. Abnormal bowel movements equals a need for more digestive enzymes.

No doctor can advise you on the exact amount of digestive enzymes, neither for the stomach (hydrochloric acid tablets), or for the pancreas you may need to take to normalize your digestion, to completely digest all your foods. Only your body knows.

In order to determine the amount of either one or types of digestive enzymes, you will have to vary the doses of one then the other, or both, up or down. This juggling may take one to two weeks before you get the right dose of each enzyme supplement and see the bowel movements perfectly normal.

Dosage requirements may vary with certain foods, stresses, moods, daily experiences and exercise.

Use this test and chart to guide you in the choice of foods that you can digest and handle well.

As long as there are any of the abnormalities indicated above, keep checking your bowel movement every time you pass one.

Make notes of changes, progress, lack of progress, both of symptoms and of the bowel movements. These should be shown to your physician during routine visits. This information can be as valuable as laboratory tests. They should be considered as lab tests.

If you are confused, or your progress is inadequate, consult with or phone your physician. Give them the information you have put together in this test.

Finally...

Reading health book after health book can be most confusing. Books can deal only in generalizations. No book knows you. No book can give you the counsel or guidelines that are perfect for you. Our bodies don't follow systems. Systems recommended for body healing must follow your body and personal individuality and needs.

You are not a theoretical human being. You are a specific, unique, mysterious, whole, complex, intricate individual. Health books should have much more meaning for you, if you clearly know everything about yourself: your heredity, biochemistry, nature, your ecology, environment and stresses, weaknesses, lifestyles, habits and excesses, your body, mind and emotions, in other words, the complete whole you.

How do all the ways that you are living, everything that you do to, and for, or against yourself; your diet, attitudes, lifework and pleasures fit with the nature of who you really are and your optimal living needs? How can you recognize, select and use from any book, only those concepts that fit your nature and your needs?

Everybody needs answers. There is one book that could provide adequate answers. That is the book entitled "YOU".

In the meantime, I hope you have found *this* book very helpful in starting your journey to optimal health!

REFERENCES

Review of Physiological Chemistry - H. A. Harper - Lange Medical Publications

Therapeutic Manual - Dr. Royal Lee, Lee Foundation for Nutritional Research, Milwaukee, Wisconsin

Pathological Physiology Mechanisms of Disease - Dr. W. Sodeman

The Illustrated Hydropathic Encyclopedia - Dr. R. T. Trall

How to Treat the Sick without Medicine - Dr. James C. Jackson

Impaired Health, Its Cause and Cure - Dr. J.H. Tilden

Toxemia, The universal Disease – Dr. J. H. Tilden

Books and articles related to liver and its functions from, *"Patient Education Publications"*(P.E.P), by the same author

The world of the Living Cell in Your Body is Immunity/Resistance G.I. [Gastro- intestinal] Detox

Pancreas – Your Biochemical Microprocessor Health Starts in the Stomach

Oils, Fats and Cholesterol

The A's, B's and 3 C's of Healthy of Healing

Choline

Proteins are for Living

High Blood Pressure Care

The Nature of Healing When Nature is Healing

Natural Pathways to Total Person Healthcare

To treat the Sick without Medicine by Dr. J.C. Jackson

Impaired Health, Its Causes and Cure by Dr. J.H. Tilden

ABOUT THE AUTHOR

Dr. Elvis Ali is highly respected for his work in Naturopathic Medicine. Dr. Elvis, as he is affectionately known, has been in private practice for over 30 years, specializing in Chinese and sports medicine and nutrition. With impressive credentials - Bachelor of Science, majoring in Biology, Licensed Acupuncturist, Doctorate in Naturopathic Medicine; Mind/Body Medicine at Harvard Medical School, Diploma in Homeopathic Medicine - he lectures internationally, written several books and appeared on radio and television shows. His passion lies in empowering people by educating them on complementary health and wellness, and non-intrusive options.

Printed in Great Britain
by Amazon